Welcome to the ***"Weight Loss Muscle Gain Cookbook: Macro Friendly Grab & Burn Fat, Build Muscles, Low, Medium, High Carb Days."*** This cookbook is designed to be your ultimate guide to achieving your fitness goals through delicious, nutritious meals tailored to support weight loss and muscle gain. Whether you're a fitness enthusiast, a seasoned athlete, or someone just starting on your health journey, this book offers a comprehensive approach to meal planning that aligns with your dietary needs and preferences.

Why This Cookbook?

Understanding the intricate balance between macronutrients—carbohydrates, proteins, and fats—is crucial for anyone looking to optimize their diet for fat loss and muscle building. This cookbook simplifies the complexity of meal planning by providing you with macro-friendly recipes that fit seamlessly into your daily routine. Our recipes are crafted to cater to different carbohydrate intake levels, including low, medium, and high carb days, ensuring that your nutritional needs are met no matter your workout schedule.

What You Will Find Inside

1. Macro-Friendly Recipes: Each recipe includes detailed macronutrient breakdowns to help you track your intake effortlessly. This allows you to enjoy meals without the stress of counting every calorie.

2. Diverse Meal Plans: The cookbook offers meal plans for various dietary preferences, including vegetarian, vegan, gluten-free, and dairy-free options, ensuring everyone can find something that suits their needs.

3. Carb Cycling Guide: Learn the benefits of carb cycling and how to implement low, medium, and high carb days into your routine to maximize fat burning and muscle building.

4. Meal Prep Tips: Practical advice on how to prepare and store meals ahead of time, making it easier to stay on track with your nutrition goals even on busy days.

5. Fitness Integration: Insights on how to align your diet with your workout regimen to enhance performance and recovery.

Embark on this culinary journey with us, and discover how delicious and fulfilling healthy eating can be. With every recipe, you are one step closer to achieving your fitness goals and leading a healthier, happier life.

I. Greek yogurt with berries and honey

Ingredient:

- 1 cup plain Greek yogurt
- 1/2 cup mixed berries (such as blueberries, raspberries, blackberries)
- 1·2 tbsp honey

Instructions:

1. Scoop the Greek yogurt into a bowl.

2. Top the yogurt with the mixed berries.

3. Drizzle the honey over the top.

This recipe provides a balance of protein, carbohydrates, and healthy fats that can support both weight loss and muscle gain goals:

- Greek yogurt is high in protein, which helps build and maintain muscle mass.

- The berries provide fiber, vitamins, and antioxidants to support overall health.

- Honey adds natural sweetness and carbohydrates to fuel your workouts.

The combination of protein·rich yogurt, fiber·filled berries, and natural sweetener makes this a nutritious and satisfying snack or light meal. Adjust the amounts of each ingredient to suit your individual calorie and macronutrient needs.

2. Scrambled eggs with spinach and mushrooms

Ingredient:

- 3 large eggs
- 1 tbsp olive oil
- 1 cup sliced mushrooms
- 1 cup fresh spinach, chopped
- 1 tbsp milk or water (optional)
- Salt and pepper to taste

Instructions:

1. Crack the eggs into a small bowl and whisk them lightly with a fork or small whisk. Add the milk or water if desired to make the eggs fluffier.

2. Heat the olive oil in a non•stick skillet over medium heat.

3. Add the sliced mushrooms and sauté for 2•3 minutes until they start to soften.

4. Add the chopped spinach and continue cooking for 1•2 minutes until the spinach is wilted.

5. Pour the whisked eggs into the skillet and use a spatula to gently push and fold the eggs as they cook, about 2•3 minutes, until the eggs are softly scrambled.

6. Season with salt and pepper to taste.

This scrambled egg dish provides a balance of protein, vegetables, and healthy fats. The spinach and mushrooms add extra nutrients and fiber. It's a quick, easy, and nutritious breakfast or anytime meal that can support both weight loss and muscle gain goals.

3. Oatmeal with almond butter and banana

Ingredient:

- 1/2 cup rolled oats
- 1 cup unsweetened almond milk (or milk of choice)
- 1 tbsp almond butter
- 1 small banana, sliced
- 1 tsp honey (optional)
- Cinnamon to taste

Instructions:

1. In a small saucepan, combine the rolled oats and almond milk. Bring to a simmer over medium heat, stirring occasionally, until the oats are cooked through and have reached your desired consistency, about 5-7 minutes.

2. Remove the oatmeal from heat and stir in the almond butter until well combined.

3. Top the oatmeal with the sliced banana. Drizzle with honey if desired and sprinkle with cinnamon.

This oatmeal dish provides a balance of complex carbs, protein, healthy fats, and fiber to support both weight loss and muscle gain:

- Oats are a complex carb that provides sustained energy and fiber to keep you feeling full.

- Almond butter adds protein and healthy monounsaturated fats to help build and maintain muscle.

- Banana provides natural sweetness, potassium, and additional carbs to fuel your workouts.

- Cinnamon and honey (optional) add flavor without extra calories.

Adjust the portions to fit your individual calorie and macronutrient needs. This makes a nutritious and satisfying breakfast or snack.

4. Cottage cheese with pineapple

Ingredient:

- 1 cup low•fat or non•fat cottage cheese
- 1/2 cup fresh pineapple chunks
- 1 tsp honey (optional)

Instructions:

1. Scoop the cottage cheese into a bowl.

2. Top the cottage cheese with the fresh pineapple chunks.

3. Drizzle the honey over the top, if desired.

This cottage cheese and pineapple dish provides a great balance of nutrients to support both weight loss and muscle gain:

Weight Loss Benefits:

- Cottage cheese is high in protein, which helps keep you feeling full and satisfied.

- Pineapple is low in calories but high in fiber, vitamins, and minerals.

- The natural sweetness from the pineapple can help curb sugar cravings.

Muscle Gain Benefits:

- The protein in cottage cheese helps build and repair muscle tissue.

- Pineapple contains bromelain, an enzyme that may aid muscle recovery.

- The carbohydrates from the pineapple provide energy to fuel your workouts.

You can adjust the portion sizes to fit your individual calorie and macronutrient needs. This makes a great snack or light meal that provides a balance of protein, carbs, and healthy nutrients.

5. Protein smoothie with spinach, banana, and protein powder

Ingredient:

- 1 cup unsweetened almond milk (or milk of choice)
- 1 cup fresh spinach
- 1 medium banana, frozen
- 1 scoop vanilla or unflavored protein powder
- 1 tbsp almond butter (optional)
- Ice cubes (optional)

Instructions:

1. Add the almond milk, spinach, banana, and protein powder to a high-powered blender.

2. Blend on high speed until smooth and creamy, about 30-60 seconds.

3. If using, add the almond butter and blend again until fully incorporated.

4. Add ice cubes if you want a thicker, colder smoothie.

This smoothie provides an excellent balance of protein, carbohydrates, healthy fats, and essential vitamins and minerals to support both weight loss and muscle gain:

Weight Loss Benefits:

- Spinach is low in calories but high in fiber, vitamins, and minerals to support overall health.
- Banana provides natural sweetness and carbohydrates to fuel your body.
- Protein powder helps keep you feeling full and satisfied.
- Almond butter adds healthy fats to promote feelings of fullness.

Muscle Gain Benefits:

- Protein powder supplies high-quality protein to help build and repair muscle tissue.
- Banana and almond butter provide carbohydrates and healthy fats to support muscle recovery.
- Spinach is rich in nutrients like magnesium and potassium that are important for muscle function.

Adjust the ingredient amounts to suit your individual calorie and macronutrient needs. This makes a nutritious and delicious smoothie that can be enjoyed as a meal replacement or snack.

6. Quinoa breakfast bowl with avocado and poached egg

Ingredient:

- 1/2 cup cooked quinoa
- 1/2 avocado, sliced
- 1 poached egg
- 1 tbsp olive oil
- Salt and pepper to taste
- Optional toppings: chopped tomatoes, sliced green onions, hot sauce

Instructions:

1. Cook the quinoa according to package instructions. Allow to cool slightly.

2. Bring a small saucepan of water to a gentle simmer. Crack the egg into the water and poach for 3•5 minutes until the white is set but the yolk is still runny.

3. Scoop the cooked quinoa into a bowl. Top with the sliced avocado and the poached egg.

4. Drizzle the olive oil over the top and season with salt and pepper. Add any additional desired toppings.

This quinoa breakfast bowl provides a balance of complex carbs, healthy fats, protein, and fiber to support both weight loss and muscle gain:

Weight Loss Benefits:
- Quinoa is a high•fiber, high•protein grain that can help keep you feeling full.
- Avocado provides heart•healthy monounsaturated fats to promote feelings of satiety.
- The poached egg adds protein to help maintain muscle mass while in a calorie deficit.

Muscle Gain Benefits:
- Quinoa is a complex carb that provides sustained energy to fuel your workouts.
- Avocado contains healthy fats that are important for hormone production and muscle recovery.
- The egg is an excellent source of high•quality protein to support muscle building and repair.

Adjust the portion sizes to fit your individual calorie and macronutrient needs. This makes a nutritious and satisfying breakfast or anytime meal.

7. Whole grain toast with avocado and smoked salmon

Ingredient:

- 2 slices whole grain bread, toasted
- 1/2 avocado, mashed or sliced
- 2•3 oz smoked salmon
- 1 tsp olive oil
- Squeeze of lemon juice
- Salt and pepper to taste
- Optional toppings: capers, red onion, dill

Instructions:

1. Toast the whole grain bread until lightly golden brown.

2. Spread the mashed or sliced avocado evenly over the toast.

3. Top the avocado with the smoked salmon.

4. Drizzle the olive oil and a squeeze of lemon juice over the top.

5. Season with salt and pepper to taste.

6. Add any optional toppings like capers, red onion, or dill.

This open•faced toast provides a balance of healthy fats, protein, and complex carbs to support both weight loss and muscle gain:

Weight Loss Benefits:
- Whole grain bread provides fiber to help keep you feeling full.
- Avocado is rich in monounsaturated fats that can promote feelings of satiety.
- Smoked salmon is a lean protein source that can help maintain muscle mass.

Muscle Gain Benefits:
- The healthy fats from the avocado and salmon support hormone production and muscle recovery.
- The protein from the salmon helps build and repair muscle tissue.
- The complex carbs from the whole grain bread provide sustained energy for workouts.

Adjust the portion sizes to fit your individual calorie and macronutrient needs. This makes a nutritious and satisfying breakfast, lunch, or snack.

8. Chia seed pudding with mixed berries

Ingredient:

- 1/4 cup chia seeds
- 1 cup unsweetened almond milk (or milk of choice)
- 1 tbsp honey (optional)
- 1/2 cup mixed berries (such as blueberries, raspberries, blackberries)

Instructions:

1. In a medium bowl, whisk together the chia seeds and almond milk until well combined.

2. Cover and refrigerate for at least 2 hours, or overnight, stirring occasionally, until the mixture has thickened to a pudding•like consistency.

3. If using, stir in the honey until fully incorporated.

4. Top the chia pudding with the mixed berries.

This chia seed pudding provides a balance of fiber, protein, healthy fats, and antioxidants to support both weight loss and muscle gain:

Weight Loss Benefits:
- Chia seeds are high in fiber, which can help keep you feeling full and satisfied.
- The protein in the chia seeds and milk can also contribute to feelings of fullness.
- Berries are low in calories but high in fiber, vitamins, and antioxidants.

Muscle Gain Benefits:
- Chia seeds contain alpha•linolenic acid, an omega•3 fatty acid that may support muscle recovery.
- The protein in the chia seeds and milk helps build and repair muscle tissue.
- Berries provide carbohydrates to fuel your workouts.

You can adjust the amount of honey or use a non•caloric sweetener if you prefer a less sweet pudding. This makes a nutritious and delicious breakfast, snack, or dessert.

9. Turkey sausage and egg white wrap

Ingredient:

- 2 egg whites
- 1 turkey sausage patty or link, cooked and crumbled
- 1 whole wheat tortilla or wrap
- 1 tbsp shredded low•fat cheddar cheese (optional)
- Salt and pepper to taste

Instructions:

1. In a small non•stick skillet, cook the egg whites over medium heat, stirring frequently, until they are set, about 2•3 minutes.

2. Remove the egg whites from the heat and stir in the crumbled turkey sausage.

3. Lay the whole wheat tortilla or wrap on a flat surface. Spoon the egg white and sausage mixture onto the center of the wrap.

4. If using, sprinkle the shredded cheese over the top.

5. Fold the bottom of the wrap up, then fold in the sides and roll up tightly.

This turkey sausage and egg white wrap provides a balance of protein, complex carbs, and healthy fats to support both weight loss and muscle gain:

Weight Loss Benefits:
- Egg whites are low in calories but high in protein to help keep you feeling full.
- Turkey sausage is a lean protein source that can help maintain muscle mass.
- The whole wheat wrap provides fiber•rich complex carbs to fuel your body.

Muscle Gain Benefits:
- The protein from the egg whites and turkey sausage supports muscle building and repair.
- The complex carbs in the whole wheat wrap provide sustained energy for your workouts.
- The wrap format makes this a portable and convenient meal or snack.

Adjust the portion sizes to fit your individual calorie and macronutrient needs. This makes a nutritious and satisfying breakfast or anytime meal.

10. Almond flour pancakes with fresh berries

Ingredient:

- 1 cup almond flour
- 2 eggs
- 1/4 cup unsweetened almond milk
- 1 tsp baking powder
- 1/2 tsp vanilla extract
- 1/4 tsp cinnamon
- 1 cup fresh berries (such as blueberries, raspberries, or a mix)
- Butter or coconut oil for cooking
- Maple syrup (optional)

Instructions:

1. In a medium bowl, whisk together the almond flour, eggs, almond milk, baking powder, vanilla, and cinnamon until a smooth batter forms.

2. Heat a non•stick skillet or griddle over medium heat and grease with a small amount of butter or coconut oil.

3. Scoop about 1/4 cup of the batter onto the hot surface and cook for 2•3 minutes per side, until golden brown.

4. Top the cooked pancakes with the fresh berries. Drizzle with a small amount of maple syrup if desired.

These almond flour pancakes provide a nutritious and delicious breakfast option that can support both weight loss and muscle gain goals:

Weight Loss Benefits:
- Almond flour is high in protein and fiber, which can help keep you feeling full.
- Berries are low in calories but high in fiber, vitamins, and antioxidants.
- The pancakes are free of added sugars, making them a healthier alternative to traditional pancakes.

Muscle Gain Benefits:
- Almond flour is a good source of healthy fats that can support muscle recovery.
- Eggs provide high•quality protein to help build and repair muscle tissue.
- The berries offer carbohydrates to fuel your workouts.

Adjust the portion sizes to fit your individual calorie and macronutrient needs. This makes a satisfying and nutritious breakfast or anytime meal.

II. Grilled chicken salad with mixed greens and balsamic vinaigrette

Ingredient:

- 4 oz grilled chicken breast, sliced
- 2 cups mixed greens (such as spinach, arugula, kale)
- 1/2 cup cherry tomatoes, halved
- 1/4 cup sliced cucumber
- 2 tbsp crumbled feta cheese (optional)
- 2 tbsp balsamic vinaigrette

For the Balsamic Vinaigrette:

- 2 tbsp balsamic vinegar
- 1 tbsp olive oil
- 1 tsp Dijon mustard
- 1 tsp honey
- Salt and pepper to taste

Instructions:

1. Make the balsamic vinaigrette by whisking together all the vinaigrette ingredients in a small bowl. Set aside.

2. In a large salad bowl, combine the mixed greens, cherry tomatoes, cucumber, and feta cheese (if using).

3. Top the salad with the grilled chicken slices. Drizzle the balsamic vinaigrette over the top and toss gently to coat.

This grilled chicken salad provides a balance of lean protein, fiber•rich greens, and healthy fats to support both weight loss and muscle gain:

Weight Loss Benefits:

- The mixed greens are low in calories but high in fiber and nutrients to keep you feeling full.
- Grilled chicken is a lean protein source that can help maintain muscle mass during weight loss.
- The balsamic vinaigrette is low in calories but adds flavor without heavy dressings.

Muscle Gain Benefits:

- The protein from the grilled chicken supports muscle building and repair.
- The healthy fats in the olive oil and vinaigrette can aid muscle recovery.
- The carbohydrates from the greens provide energy to fuel your workouts.

12. Quinoa and black bean bowl with avocado and salsa

Ingredient:

- 1/2 cup cooked quinoa
- 1/2 cup canned black beans, rinsed and drained
- 1/2 avocado, diced
- 1/4 cup fresh salsa
- 1 tbsp lime juice
- Salt and pepper to taste
- Optional toppings: chopped cilantro, diced red onion, hot sauce

Instructions:

1. In a medium bowl, combine the cooked quinoa and black beans.

2. Top with the diced avocado and salsa.

3. Drizzle the lime juice over the top and season with salt and pepper.

4. Add any optional toppings like cilantro, red onion, or hot sauce.

This quinoa and black bean bowl provides a balance of complex carbs, protein, healthy fats, and fiber to support both weight loss and muscle gain:

Weight Loss Benefits:
- Quinoa is a high•fiber, high•protein grain that can help keep you feeling full.
- Black beans are a great source of plant•based protein and fiber.
- Avocado provides heart•healthy monounsaturated fats to promote feelings of satiety.
- Salsa adds flavor without a lot of extra calories.

Muscle Gain Benefits:
- The protein from the quinoa and black beans supports muscle building and repair.
- Avocado contains healthy fats that are important for hormone production and muscle recovery.
- The complex carbs in the quinoa provide sustained energy to fuel your workouts.

Adjust the portion sizes to fit your individual calorie and macronutrient needs. This makes a nutritious and satisfying meal or snack.

13. Turkey and avocado lettuce wrap

Ingredient:

- 3-4 oz sliced turkey breast
- 1/2 avocado, sliced
- 2-3 large lettuce leaves (such as romaine or butter lettuce)
- 1 tbsp hummus or tzatziki sauce (optional)
- Salt and pepper to taste

Instructions:

1. Lay the lettuce leaves flat on a clean surface.

2. Layer the sliced turkey breast evenly over the lettuce leaves.

3. Top the turkey with the sliced avocado.

4. If using, spread a thin layer of hummus or tzatziki sauce over the avocado.

5. Season with salt and pepper to taste.

6. Carefully roll up the lettuce leaves around the fillings to create your wrap.

This turkey and avocado lettuce wrap provides a balance of lean protein, healthy fats, and fiber to support both weight loss and muscle gain:

Weight Loss Benefits:
- Turkey breast is a lean protein source that can help keep you feeling full and satisfied.
- Avocado provides heart-healthy monounsaturated fats to promote feelings of fullness.
- Lettuce leaves are low in calories but high in fiber and nutrients.

Muscle Gain Benefits:
- The protein from the turkey supports muscle building and repair.
- Avocado contains healthy fats that are important for hormone production and muscle recovery.
- The wrap format makes this a portable and convenient meal or snack.

Adjust the portion sizes to fit your individual calorie and macronutrient needs. You can also experiment with different protein sources, vegetables, and condiments to customize this recipe to your taste preferences.

14. Tuna salad with celery and Greek yogurt

Ingredient:

- 5 oz canned tuna, drained
- 1/4 cup plain Greek yogurt
- 1 stalk celery, diced
- 1 tbsp diced red onion (optional)
- 1 tsp Dijon mustard
- 1 tsp lemon juice
- Salt and pepper to taste

Instructions:

1. In a medium bowl, combine the drained tuna, Greek yogurt, diced celery, red onion (if using), Dijon mustard, and lemon juice.

2. Mix all the ingredients together until well combined.

3. Season with salt and pepper to taste.

This tuna salad provides a balance of protein, healthy fats, and fiber to support both weight loss and muscle gain:

Weight Loss Benefits:
- Tuna is a lean protein source that can help keep you feeling full and satisfied.
- Greek yogurt adds creaminess and extra protein without a lot of calories.
- Celery is low in calories but high in fiber to promote feelings of fullness.

Muscle Gain Benefits:
- The protein from the tuna and Greek yogurt supports muscle building and repair.
- The healthy fats from the tuna can aid muscle recovery.
- The recipe is versatile and can be enjoyed on its own, on top of greens, or as a sandwich filling.

Adjust the portion sizes to fit your individual calorie and macronutrient needs. This makes a nutritious and delicious snack or light meal.

15. Lentil soup with kale

Ingredient:

- 1 cup dry brown or green lentils, rinsed
- 4 cups low•sodium vegetable or chicken broth
- 1 tbsp olive oil
- 1 onion, diced
- 3 cloves garlic, minced
- 2 carrots, peeled and diced
- 2 stalks celery, diced
- 1 tsp ground cumin
- 1 tsp dried oregano
- 1/4 tsp red pepper flakes (optional)
- 4 cups chopped kale, stems removed
- Salt and pepper to taste

Instructions:

1. In a large pot, bring the lentils and broth to a boil over high heat. Reduce heat to medium•low, cover, and simmer for 15•20 minutes, until lentils are tender.

2. In a separate skillet, heat the olive oil over medium heat. Add the onion, garlic, carrots, and celery. Sauté for 5•7 minutes until vegetables are softened.

3. Add the sautéed vegetables, cumin, oregano, and red pepper flakes (if using) to the pot with the cooked lentils. Stir to combine.

4. Add the chopped kale and continue simmering for 5•10 minutes, until the kale is wilted and tender. Season with salt and pepper to taste.

This lentil and kale soup provides a nutritious balance of plant•based protein, fiber, and essential vitamins and minerals to support both weight loss and muscle gain:

Weight Loss Benefits:
- Lentils are high in fiber and protein, which can help keep you feeling full.
- Kale is low in calories but packed with nutrients like vitamins A, C, and K.
- The soup format makes this a satisfying and hydrating meal.

Muscle Gain Benefits:
- The protein from the lentils supports muscle building and repair.
- Kale is rich in antioxidants that may aid muscle recovery.
- The complex carbs from the lentils and vegetables provide sustained energy.

16. Baked salmon with quinoa and steamed broccoli

Ingredient:

- 4 oz salmon fillet
- 1/2 cup cooked quinoa
- 1 cup broccoli florets, steamed
- 1 tsp olive oil
- 1 tbsp lemon juice
- Salt and pepper to taste

Instructions:

1. Preheat your oven to 400°F (200°C).

2. Place the salmon fillet on a baking sheet lined with parchment paper or foil. Drizzle with 1 tsp of olive oil and season with salt and pepper.

3. Bake the salmon for 12•15 minutes, or until it flakes easily with a fork.

4. While the salmon is baking, cook the quinoa according to package instructions.

5. Steam the broccoli florets until tender, about 5•7 minutes.

6. Once the salmon is cooked, flake it into chunks with a fork.

7. Arrange the baked salmon, cooked quinoa, and steamed broccoli on a plate. Drizzle the salmon with 1 tbsp of lemon juice.

This baked salmon, quinoa, and broccoli dish provides a balanced meal that can support both weight loss and muscle gain:

Weight Loss Benefits:
- Salmon is a lean protein source that can help keep you feeling full and satisfied.
- Quinoa is a high•fiber, high•protein grain that can also contribute to feelings of fullness.
- Broccoli is low in calories but high in fiber, vitamins, and minerals.

Muscle Gain Benefits:
- The protein from the salmon and quinoa supports muscle building and repair.
- The healthy fats in the salmon can aid muscle recovery.
- The complex carbs from the quinoa and broccoli provide sustained energy to fuel your workouts.

17. Chicken and vegetable stir·fry with brown rice

Ingredient:

• 4 oz boneless, skinless chicken breast, cut into bite·sized pieces
• 1 cup mixed vegetables (such as broccoli, bell peppers, snap peas, carrots)
• 1/2 cup cooked brown rice
• 1 tbsp low·sodium soy sauce or tamari
• 1 tsp sesame oil
• 1 tsp minced garlic
• 1 tsp minced ginger
• Salt and pepper to taste

Instructions:

1. Cook the brown rice according to package instructions.

2. In a large skillet or wok, heat the sesame oil over medium·high heat.

3. Add the chicken and stir·fry for 3·4 minutes until lightly browned.

4. Add the mixed vegetables, garlic, and ginger. Stir·fry for an additional 5·7 minutes until the vegetables are tender·crisp.

5. Pour in the soy sauce or tamari and stir to coat the chicken and vegetables.

6. Serve the stir·fry over the cooked brown rice. Season with salt and pepper to taste.

This chicken and vegetable stir·fry with brown rice provides a balance of lean protein, complex carbs, and fiber·rich vegetables to support both weight loss and muscle gain:

Weight Loss Benefits:
• Chicken breast is a lean protein source that can help keep you feeling full.
• The mixed vegetables are low in calories but high in fiber, vitamins, and minerals.
• Brown rice is a complex carb that provides sustained energy without blood sugar spikes.

Muscle Gain Benefits:
• The protein from the chicken supports muscle building and repair.
• The complex carbs in the brown rice provide fuel for your workouts.
• The vegetables offer antioxidants and other nutrients that may aid muscle recovery.

18. Greek salad with grilled shrimp

Ingredient:

- 4 oz grilled shrimp
- 2 cups mixed greens (such as romaine, spinach, arugula)
- 1/2 cup diced cucumber
- 1/4 cup diced tomatoes
- 2 tbsp crumbled feta cheese
- 1 tbsp sliced kalamata olives
- 1 tbsp olive oil
- 1 tbsp red wine vinegar
- 1 tsp dried oregano
- Salt and pepper to taste

Instructions:

1. Preheat your grill or grill pan to medium•high heat. Grill the shrimp for 2•3 minutes per side, until opaque and cooked through. Set aside.

2. In a large salad bowl, combine the mixed greens, cucumber, tomatoes, feta cheese, and olives.

3. In a small bowl, whisk together the olive oil, red wine vinegar, and dried oregano to make the dressing.

4. Drizzle the dressing over the salad and toss gently to coat. Top the salad with the grilled shrimp. Season with salt and pepper to taste.

This Greek salad with grilled shrimp provides a balance of lean protein, healthy fats, and fiber•rich vegetables to support both weight loss and muscle gain:

Weight Loss Benefits:
- Shrimp is a lean protein source that can help keep you feeling full and satisfied.
- The mixed greens, cucumber, and tomatoes are low in calories but high in fiber and nutrients.
- The olive oil and vinegar dressing adds flavor without a lot of extra calories.

Muscle Gain Benefits:
- The protein from the shrimp supports muscle building and repair.
- The healthy fats in the olive oil can aid muscle recovery.
- The salad format makes this a light yet satisfying meal.

19. Turkey chili with kidney beans

Ingredient:

- 1 lb ground turkey
- 1 onion, diced
- 3 cloves garlic, minced
- 1 bell pepper, diced
- 2 cans (15 oz each) kidney beans, rinsed and drained
- 1 can (28 oz) diced tomatoes
- 2 tbsp chili powder
- 1 tsp ground cumin
- 1 tsp dried oregano
- 1/4 tsp cayenne pepper (optional)
- Salt and pepper to taste
- Chopped cilantro for garnish (optional)

Instructions:

1. In a large pot or Dutch oven, cook the ground turkey over medium·high heat, breaking it up with a wooden spoon, until browned, about 5·7 minutes.

2. Add the diced onion, garlic, and bell pepper. Sauté for 3·4 minutes until the vegetables are softened.

3. Stir in the kidney beans, diced tomatoes, chili powder, cumin, oregano, and cayenne (if using). Season with salt and pepper.

4. Bring the chili to a simmer, then reduce heat to medium·low and let it cook for 20·25 minutes, stirring occasionally, until the flavors have melded. Serve the turkey chili hot, garnished with chopped cilantro if desired.

This turkey chili with kidney beans provides a balance of lean protein, complex carbs, and fiber to support both weight loss and muscle gain:

Weight Loss Benefits:

- Ground turkey is a lean protein source that can help keep you feeling full.
- Kidney beans are high in fiber, which can also contribute to feelings of fullness.
- The chili format makes this a satisfying and nutrient·dense meal.

Muscle Gain Benefits:

- The protein from the turkey supports muscle building and repair.
- The complex carbs from the beans provide sustained energy to fuel your workouts.
- The chili is packed with vitamins, minerals, and antioxidants that may aid muscle recovery

20. Chickpea and cucumber salad with lemon dressing

Ingredient:

- 1 (15 oz) can chickpeas, rinsed and drained
- 1 cup diced cucumber
- 1/4 cup diced red onion
- 2 tbsp chopped fresh parsley
- 2 tbsp olive oil
- 2 tbsp lemon juice
- 1 tsp Dijon mustard
- 1 tsp honey
- Salt and pepper to taste

Instructions:

1. In a large bowl, combine the rinsed and drained chickpeas, diced cucumber, red onion, and chopped parsley.

2. In a small bowl, whisk together the olive oil, lemon juice, Dijon mustard, and honey to make the dressing.

3. Pour the dressing over the chickpea and cucumber mixture and toss gently to coat.

4. Season with salt and pepper to taste. Refrigerate the salad for at least 30 minutes to allow the flavors to meld.

This chickpea and cucumber salad provides a balance of plant·based protein, fiber, and healthy fats to support both weight loss and muscle gain:

Weight Loss Benefits:
- Chickpeas are high in fiber and protein, which can help keep you feeling full.
- Cucumbers are low in calories but high in water content to help with hydration.
- The lemon dressing adds flavor without a lot of extra calories.

Muscle Gain Benefits:
- The protein from the chickpeas supports muscle building and repair.
- The healthy fats in the olive oil can aid muscle recovery.
- The salad format makes this a light yet satisfying meal or snack.

Adjust the portion sizes to fit your individual calorie and macronutrient needs. This makes a nutritious and refreshing side dish or light main course.

21. Grilled steak with sweet potato and asparagus

Ingredient:

- 6 oz grilled steak (such as flank or sirloin)
- 1 medium sweet potato, cubed and roasted
- 1 cup asparagus spears, steamed
- 1 tbsp olive oil
- Salt and pepper to taste

Instructions:

1. Preheat your grill or grill pan to medium•high heat.

2. Season the steak with salt and pepper on both sides.

3. Grill the steak for 3•5 minutes per side, depending on thickness, until it reaches your desired doneness. Let the steak rest for 5 minutes before slicing.

4. While the steak is cooking, roast the cubed sweet potato in the oven at 400°F (200°C) for 20•25 minutes, until tender.

5. Steam the asparagus spears for 5•7 minutes, until bright green and tender•crisp.

6. Arrange the grilled steak, roasted sweet potato, and steamed asparagus on a plate.

7. Drizzle the entire dish with 1 tbsp of olive oil.

This grilled steak, sweet potato, and asparagus meal provides a balance of lean protein, complex carbs, and fiber•rich vegetables to support both weight loss and muscle gain:

Weight Loss Benefits:
- Steak is a lean protein source that can help keep you feeling full and satisfied.
- Sweet potato is a complex carb that provides sustained energy without blood sugar spikes.
- Asparagus is low in calories but high in fiber, vitamins, and minerals.

Muscle Gain Benefits:
- The protein from the steak supports muscle building and repair.
- The complex carbs in the sweet potato provide fuel for your workouts.
- The healthy fats from the olive oil can aid muscle recovery.

22. Baked cod with roasted Brussels sprouts

Ingredient:

- 6 oz cod fillet
- 1 lb Brussels sprouts, trimmed and halved
- 1 tbsp olive oil
- 1 tsp garlic powder
- Salt and pepper to taste

Instructions:

1. Preheat your oven to 400°F (200°C).

2. In a large baking dish or sheet pan, toss the trimmed and halved Brussels sprouts with 1 tbsp of olive oil, garlic powder, salt, and pepper.

3. Roast the Brussels sprouts for 15•20 minutes, stirring halfway, until they are tender and lightly browned.

4. While the Brussels sprouts are roasting, place the cod fillet on a separate baking sheet or in a baking dish. Season the cod with salt and pepper.

5. Bake the cod for 12•15 minutes, or until it flakes easily with a fork.

6. Serve the baked cod alongside the roasted Brussels sprouts.

This baked cod and roasted Brussels sprouts dish provides a balance of lean protein, fiber•rich vegetables, and healthy fats to support both weight loss and muscle gain:

Weight Loss Benefits:
- Cod is a lean, low•calorie protein source that can help keep you feeling full.
- Brussels sprouts are low in calories but high in fiber, vitamins, and minerals.
- The baking method avoids the need for added oils or heavy sauces.

Muscle Gain Benefits:
- The protein from the cod supports muscle building and repair.
- The healthy fats in the olive oil can aid muscle recovery.
- The complex carbs and fiber from the Brussels sprouts provide sustained energy.

Adjust the portion sizes to fit your individual calorie and macronutrient needs. This makes a nutritious and satisfying meal.

23. Spaghetti squash with turkey meatballs

Ingredient:

For the Spaghetti Squash:
• 1 medium spaghetti squash, halved lengthwise and seeds removed
• 1 tbsp olive oil
• Salt and pepper to taste

For the Turkey Meatballs:
• 1 lb ground turkey
• 1/2 cup whole wheat breadcrumbs
• 1 egg
• 2 tbsp grated Parmesan cheese
• 2 cloves garlic, minced
• 1 tsp dried oregano
• 1/4 tsp red pepper flakes (optional)
• Salt and pepper to taste

Instructions:

1. Preheat your oven to 400°F (200°C).

2. Place the spaghetti squash halves cut•side up on a baking sheet. Drizzle with 1 tbsp of olive oil and season with salt and pepper.

3. Roast the spaghetti squash for 40•50 minutes, until tender when pierced with a fork.

4. While the squash is roasting, prepare the turkey meatballs. In a large bowl, combine the ground turkey, breadcrumbs, egg, Parmesan, garlic, oregano, and red pepper flakes (if using). Season with salt and pepper.

5. Roll the mixture into 1•inch meatballs and place them on a separate baking sheet.

6. Bake the meatballs for 18•20 minutes, until cooked through.

7. Once the spaghetti squash is tender, use a fork to gently scrape the flesh into strands. Serve the spaghetti squash "noodles" topped with the baked turkey meatballs.

Adjust the portion sizes to fit your individual calorie and macronutrient needs. This makes a nutritious and satisfying meal.

24. Chicken fajitas with bell peppers and onions

Ingredient:

- 6 oz boneless, skinless chicken breast, sliced into strips
- 1 red bell pepper, sliced
- 1 green bell pepper, sliced
- 1 onion, sliced
- 1 tbsp olive oil
- 1 tsp chili powder
- 1 tsp cumin
- 1/2 tsp garlic powder
- Salt and pepper to taste
- 4 small whole wheat tortillas or lettuce wraps

Instructions:

1. In a large skillet or wok, heat the olive oil over medium•high heat.

2. Add the sliced chicken, bell peppers, and onions to the skillet. Season with the chili powder, cumin, garlic powder, salt, and pepper.

3. Stir•fry the mixture for 8•10 minutes, until the chicken is cooked through and the vegetables are tender•crisp. Serve the chicken fajita mixture in the whole wheat tortillas or lettuce wraps.

This chicken fajita dish provides a balance of lean protein, fiber•rich vegetables, and complex carbs to support both weight loss and muscle gain:

Weight Loss Benefits:
- Chicken breast is a lean protein source that can help keep you feeling full.
- Bell peppers and onions are low in calories but high in fiber, vitamins, and minerals.
- Whole wheat tortillas or lettuce wraps provide complex carbs without excess calories.

Muscle Gain Benefits:
- The protein from the chicken supports muscle building and repair.
- The complex carbs from the tortillas or lettuce provide sustained energy to fuel your workouts.
- The vegetables offer antioxidants and other nutrients that may aid muscle recovery.

Adjust the portion sizes to fit your individual calorie and macronutrient needs. You can also experiment with different vegetable combinations or serve the fajita mixture over a bed of greens for a lower•carb option.

25. Beef and vegetable stew

Ingredient:

- 1 lb beef stew meat, cut into 1·inch cubes
- 2 tbsp olive oil
- 1 onion, diced
- 3 cloves garlic, minced
- 2 carrots, peeled and diced
- 2 celery stalks, diced
- 1 cup diced potatoes
- 1 cup diced butternut squash
- 4 cups low·sodium beef broth
- 1 (14.5 oz) can diced tomatoes
- 2 tsp dried thyme
- 1 bay leaf
- Salt and pepper to taste
- Chopped parsley for garnish (optional)

Instructions:

1. In a large pot or Dutch oven, heat the olive oil over medium·high heat. Add the beef cubes and brown on all sides, about 5 minutes total. Remove the beef from the pot and set aside.

2. Add the diced onion, garlic, carrots, and celery to the pot. Sauté for 5·7 minutes until the vegetables are softened.

3. Add the diced potatoes, butternut squash, beef broth, diced tomatoes, thyme, and bay leaf. Stir to combine.

4. Return the browned beef cubes to the pot and bring the stew to a boil.

5. Reduce the heat to low, cover, and simmer for 45·60 minutes, until the beef and vegetables are tender.

6. Season the stew with salt and pepper to taste. Serve the beef and vegetable stew hot, garnished with chopped parsley if desired.

Adjust the portion sizes to fit your individual calorie and macronutrient needs. This makes a nutritious and comforting meal.

26. Shrimp stir·fry with snap peas and brown rice

Ingredient:

- 8 oz raw shrimp, peeled and deveined
- 1 cup snap peas, trimmed
- 1 red bell pepper, sliced
- 1 tbsp sesame oil
- 2 tbsp low·sodium soy sauce or tamari
- 1 tsp honey
- 1 tsp grated ginger
- 2 cloves garlic, minced
- 1/4 tsp red pepper flakes (optional)
- 1 cup cooked brown rice

Instructions:

1. Cook the brown rice according to package instructions.

2. In a large skillet or wok, heat the sesame oil over medium·high heat.

3. Add the shrimp, snap peas, and bell pepper. Stir·fry for 3·4 minutes until the shrimp is opaque and the vegetables are tender·crisp.

4. In a small bowl, whisk together the soy sauce, honey, ginger, garlic, and red pepper flakes (if using).

5. Pour the sauce into the skillet and toss everything together to coat. Serve the shrimp stir·fry over the cooked brown rice.

This shrimp stir·fry with snap peas and brown rice provides a balance of lean protein, complex carbs, and fiber·rich vegetables to support both weight loss and muscle gain:

Weight Loss Benefits:

- Shrimp is a lean protein source that can help keep you feeling full.
- Snap peas and bell peppers are low in calories but high in fiber and nutrients.
- Brown rice is a complex carb that provides sustained energy without blood sugar spikes.

Muscle Gain Benefits:

- The protein from the shrimp supports muscle building and repair.
- The complex carbs in the brown rice provide fuel for your workouts.
- The vegetables offer antioxidants and other nutrients that may aid muscle recovery

27. Turkey and vegetable stuffed bell peppers

Ingredient:

- 4 bell peppers, halved lengthwise and seeds removed
- 1 lb ground turkey
- 1 cup diced onion
- 2 cloves garlic, minced
- 1 cup diced zucchini
- 1 cup diced tomatoes
- 1/2 cup cooked brown rice
- 1 tsp dried oregano
- 1/2 tsp chili powder
- Salt and pepper to taste
- 1/4 cup shredded low·fat cheddar cheese (optional)

Instructions:

1. Preheat your oven to 375°F (190°C).

2. Place the bell pepper halves in a baking dish and set aside.

3. In a large skillet over medium heat, cook the ground turkey, onion, and garlic until the turkey is browned and the vegetables are softened, about 5·7 minutes.

4. Stir in the diced zucchini, tomatoes, cooked brown rice, oregano, chili powder, salt, and pepper. Cook for an additional 2·3 minutes.

5. Spoon the turkey and vegetable mixture evenly into the bell pepper halves.

6. If using, sprinkle the shredded cheddar cheese over the top of the stuffed peppers
.

7. Bake the stuffed peppers for 20·25 minutes, until the peppers are tender and the filling is hot.

This turkey and vegetable stuffed bell pepper dish provides a balance of lean protein, complex carbs, fiber, and nutrients to support both weight loss and muscle gain:

Adjust the portion sizes to fit your individual calorie and macronutrient needs. This makes a nutritious and satisfying meal.

28. Grilled pork chops with cauliflower mash

Ingredient:

For the Pork Chops:
- 4 (4 oz) boneless pork chops
- 1 tbsp olive oil
- Salt and pepper to taste

For the Cauliflower Mash:
- 1 head of cauliflower, cut into florets
- 2 tbsp unsweetened almond milk
- 1 tbsp grated Parmesan cheese
- 1 clove garlic, minced
- Salt and pepper to taste

Instructions:

1. Preheat your grill or grill pan to medium•high heat.

2. Brush the pork chops with olive oil and season with salt and pepper.

3. Grill the pork chops for 4•5 minutes per side, until cooked through.

4. While the pork chops are grilling, bring a large pot of water to a boil. Add the cauliflower florets and cook for 8•10 minutes, until very tender.

5. Drain the cooked cauliflower and transfer it to a food processor or blender. Add the almond milk, Parmesan cheese, and garlic. Blend until smooth and creamy.

6. Season the cauliflower mash with salt and pepper to taste.

7. Serve the grilled pork chops alongside the cauliflower mash.

This grilled pork chop and cauliflower mash dish provides a balance of lean protein, healthy fats, and low•carb vegetables to support both weight loss and muscle gain:

Weight Loss Benefits:
- Pork chops are a lean protein source that can help keep you feeling full.
- Cauliflower is low in calories but high in fiber and nutrients.
- The grilling and mashing methods avoid the need for added oils or heavy saucess

Adjust the portion sizes to fit your individual calorie and macronutrient needs. This makes a nutritious and satisfying meal.

29. Baked tofu with quinoa and steamed green beans

Ingredient:

- 1 block of extra•firm tofu, pressed and cubed
- 2 tbsp soy sauce or tamari
- 1 tbsp maple syrup
- 1 tsp sesame oil
- 1 cup quinoa, cooked according to package instructions
- 1 lb green beans, trimmed and steamed

For the Tofu Marinade:

- 2 tbsp soy sauce or tamari
- 1 tbsp rice vinegar
- 1 tsp sesame oil
- 1 tsp grated ginger
- 1 clove garlic, minced

Instructions:

1. Preheat the oven to 400°F (200°C).

2. In a shallow dish, combine the tofu cubes, 2 tbsp soy sauce, 1 tbsp maple syrup, and 1 tsp sesame oil. Toss to coat the tofu evenly. Let marinate for 15•20 minutes.

3. Arrange the marinated tofu cubes on a parchment•lined baking sheet. Bake for 20•25 minutes, flipping halfway, until the tofu is crispy and golden brown.

4. While the tofu is baking, prepare the quinoa according to package instructions.

5. Steam the green beans until tender•crisp, about 5•7 minutes.

6. Serve the baked tofu over the cooked quinoa, accompanied by the steamed green beans.

This dish is a great source of plant•based protein from the tofu and quinoa, as well as fiber and nutrients from the green beans. The combination of macronutrients can support both weight loss and muscle gain goals when paired with an overall balanced diet and exercise routine.

30. Lemon herb chicken with roasted zucchini

Ingredient:

• 4 boneless, skinless chicken breasts
• 2 tbsp olive oil
• 2 tbsp lemon juice
• 1 tbsp dried oregano
• 1 tbsp dried basil
• 1 tsp garlic powder
• Salt and pepper to taste
• 2 medium zucchini, sliced into 1/2•inch rounds
• 1 tbsp olive oil
• Salt and pepper to taste

Instructions:

1. Preheat the oven to 400°F (200°C).

2. In a shallow dish, combine the olive oil, lemon juice, oregano, basil, garlic powder, salt, and pepper. Add the chicken breasts and turn to coat them evenly with the marinade. Let the chicken marinate for 15•20 minutes.

3. Arrange the marinated chicken breasts on a baking sheet.

4. In a separate bowl, toss the zucchini slices with 1 tbsp of olive oil, salt, and pepper.

5. Arrange the zucchini slices on a separate baking sheet.

6. Bake the chicken and zucchini for 20•25 minutes, or until the chicken is cooked through and the zucchini is tender and lightly browned.

7. Serve the lemon herb chicken with the roasted zucchini.

This dish is a great source of lean protein from the chicken, as well as fiber and nutrients from the zucchini. The combination of macronutrients can support both weight loss and muscle gain goals when paired with an overall balanced diet and exercise routine.

31. Apple slices with almond butter

Ingredient:

- 1 medium apple, cored and sliced
- 2•3 tbsp natural almond butter

Instructions:

1. Wash and slice the apple into thin, even slices. Remove the core.

2. Arrange the apple slices on a plate or platter.

3. Spoon the almond butter onto the apple slices, using about 1•2 teaspoons of almond butter per slice.

4. Serve immediately.

This snack is a great option for weight loss and muscle gain for a few reasons:

1. Apples are a low•calorie, high•fiber fruit that can help keep you feeling full and satisfied.

2. Almond butter provides healthy fats, protein, and fiber, which can also contribute to feelings of fullness.

3. The combination of the crisp apple and creamy almond butter makes for a delicious and nutritious snack.

4. This snack is easy to prepare and portable, making it a great option for a quick, healthy pick•me•up.

The healthy fats, fiber, and protein in this snack can help support both weight loss and muscle gain goals when incorporated into an overall balanced diet and exercise routine.

32. Greek yogurt with honey and walnuts

Ingredient:

- 1 cup plain Greek yogurt
- 1•2 tbsp honey
- 2 tbsp chopped walnuts

Instructions:

1. Scoop the Greek yogurt into a bowl.

2. Drizzle the honey over the yogurt, using 1•2 tablespoons depending on your desired sweetness level.

3. Sprinkle the chopped walnuts over the top of the honey•sweetened yogurt.

4. Serve immediately.

This snack or light meal is a great option for weight loss and muscle gain for several reasons:

1. Greek yogurt is high in protein, which can help support muscle growth and maintenance.

2. Honey provides a natural source of carbohydrates, which can help replenish glycogen stores and provide energy.

3. Walnuts are a good source of healthy fats, fiber, and protein, which can help keep you feeling full and satisfied.

4. The combination of the creamy yogurt, sweet honey, and crunchy walnuts creates a delicious and nutritious treat.

This snack is easy to prepare, portable, and can be enjoyed as a healthy breakfast, snack, or light dessert. When incorporated into an overall balanced diet and exercise routine, the nutrients in this dish can support both weight loss and muscle gain goals.

33. Carrot sticks with hummus

Ingredient:

• 2•3 medium carrots, peeled and cut into sticks
• 1/2 cup hummus (store•bought or homemade)

Instructions:

1. Wash and peel the carrots. Cut them into long, thin sticks, about 4•5 inches long.

2. Scoop the hummus into a small bowl or ramekin.

3. Arrange the carrot sticks around the hummus, allowing people to dip the carrots into the hummus.

This snack is a great choice for weight loss and muscle gain for several reasons:

1. Carrots are low in calories, high in fiber, and rich in vitamins and minerals like beta•carotene. They can help you feel full and satisfied without consuming a lot of calories.

2. Hummus is a great source of plant•based protein, healthy fats, and complex carbohydrates. The protein and healthy fats can help support muscle growth and maintenance.

3. The combination of the crunchy carrots and creamy hummus provides a satisfying and nutrient•dense snack that can curb hunger and cravings.

4. This snack is easy to prepare, portable, and can be enjoyed as a healthy mid•day or post•workout snack.

When incorporated into an overall balanced diet and exercise routine, this simple snack can support both weight loss and muscle gain goals. The fiber, protein, and healthy fats can help keep you feeling full and satisfied, while also providing the nutrients your body needs to perform and recover.

34. Hard·boiled eggs

Ingredient:

• Large eggs

Instructions:

1. Place the eggs in a single layer in a saucepan and cover with cold water by 1 inch.

2. Bring the water to a boil over high heat.

3. Once the water reaches a rolling boil, remove the pan from the heat and cover with a lid.

4. Let the eggs sit in the hot water for the following times:
   • For soft·boiled eggs: 6·7 minutes
   • For hard·boiled eggs: 12 minutes
5. Drain the hot water and cover the eggs with cold water to stop the cooking process.

6. Peel the eggs and enjoy!

Hard·boiled eggs are a great snack option for both weight loss and muscle gain for several reasons:

1. Eggs are an excellent source of high·quality protein, which is essential for building and maintaining muscle mass.

2. They are low in calories and carbohydrates, making them a great choice for weight loss.

3. Eggs are rich in nutrients like vitamins A, D, B12, and choline, which are important for overall health and well·being.

4. Hard·boiled eggs are easy to prepare, portable, and can be enjoyed as a quick, on·the·go snack.

When incorporated into an overall balanced diet and exercise routine, hard·boiled eggs can be a valuable addition to support both weight loss and muscle gain goals. The protein and nutrients in eggs can help keep you feeling full and satisfied, while also providing the building blocks your body needs to perform and recover.

35. Cottage cheese with sliced peaches

Ingredient:

• 1 cup low•fat or non•fat cottage cheese
• 1 medium peach, sliced

Instructions:
1. Scoop the cottage cheese into a bowl or container.

2. Arrange the sliced peaches on top of the cottage cheese.

This snack is an excellent choice for weight loss and muscle gain for several reasons:

1. Cottage cheese is a great source of high•quality protein, which is essential for building and maintaining muscle mass.

2. Peaches are a low•calorie, high•fiber fruit that can help you feel full and satisfied without consuming a lot of calories.

3. The combination of the creamy cottage cheese and sweet, juicy peaches provides a delicious and nutrient•dense snack.

4. This snack is easy to prepare, portable, and can be enjoyed as a healthy mid•day or post•workout treat.

When incorporated into an overall balanced diet and exercise routine, this snack can support both weight loss and muscle gain goals. The protein from the cottage cheese can help support muscle growth and maintenance, while the fiber and natural sweetness from the peaches can help curb hunger and cravings.

Additionally, cottage cheese is a versatile ingredient that can be used in a variety of recipes, making it a great addition to a healthy, balanced diet. Whether you're looking to lose weight or build muscle, this simple snack can be a valuable part of your nutrition plan.

36. Edamame with sea salt

Ingredient:

- 1 cup frozen edamame, in the pod
- 1/4 teaspoon sea salt

Instructions:

1. Bring a medium pot of water to a boil.

2. Add the frozen edamame pods and cook for 5•7 minutes, or until the pods are bright green and tender.

3. Drain the edamame and transfer to a serving bowl.

4. Sprinkle the sea salt over the edamame and toss to coat evenly.

5. Serve warm or at room temperature.

Edamame is an excellent snack choice for both weight loss and muscle gain for several reasons:

1. Edamame is a great source of plant•based protein, which is essential for building and maintaining muscle mass.

2. It's low in calories and high in fiber, making it a filling and satisfying snack that can help with weight management.

3. Edamame is rich in vitamins, minerals, and antioxidants, such as vitamin K, folate, and vitamin C, which are important for overall health and well•being.

4. The simple preparation and portability of edamame make it a convenient and easy•to•enjoy snack.

When incorporated into an overall balanced diet and exercise routine, edamame with sea salt can be a valuable addition to support both weight loss and muscle gain goals. The protein, fiber, and nutrients in edamame can help keep you feeling full and satisfied, while also providing the building blocks your body needs to perform and recover.

37. Protein bars (low sugar)

Ingredient:

- 1 cup rolled oats
- 1/2 cup unsweetened shredded coconut
- 1/2 cup almond flour
- 1/4 cup unflavored whey protein powder
- 1/4 cup unsweetened applesauce
- 1/4 cup natural peanut butter (or other nut butter)
- 2 tbsp honey
- 1 tsp vanilla extract
- 1/4 tsp salt

Instructions:

1. Preheat oven to 350°F. Line an 8x8 inch baking pan with parchment paper.

2. In a large bowl, mix together the rolled oats, shredded coconut, almond flour, and whey protein powder.

3. In a separate bowl, combine the applesauce, peanut butter, honey, vanilla, and salt. Mix well until fully incorporated.

4. Add the wet ingredients to the dry ingredients and stir until a thick dough forms.

5. Press the dough evenly into the prepared baking pan.

6. Bake for 15•18 minutes, until lightly golden on top.

7. Allow to cool completely in the pan before cutting into bars.

8. Store the protein bars in an airtight container in the refrigerator for up to 1 week.

Enjoy these low•sugar, high•protein snack bars! Let me know if you have any other questions.

38. Mixed nuts and seeds

Ingredient:

- 1 cup raw almonds
- 1/2 cup raw cashews
- 1/2 cup raw pumpkin seeds (pepitas)
- 1/2 cup raw sunflower seeds
- 1/4 cup raw walnuts
- 1/4 cup raw pecans
- 1 tsp ground cinnamon (optional)
- 1/4 tsp sea salt (optional)

Instructions:

1. In a large bowl, combine all the nuts and seeds.

2. If using, sprinkle the cinnamon and salt over the nut and seed mixture and stir to coat evenly.

3. Transfer the mixed nuts and seeds to an airtight container or resealable bag.

4. Store at room temperature for up to 2 weeks.

Variations:
- You can use any combination of raw, unsalted nuts and seeds that you prefer.
- For a little extra flavor, you can toast the nuts and seeds in a dry skillet for 2•3 minutes before mixing.
- Add a drizzle of honey or maple syrup for a lightly sweetened version.
- Toss in some dried fruit like cranberries or apricots.

This makes a great portable, protein•rich snack. The mix of nuts and seeds provides a variety of healthy fats, fiber, and nutrients. Enjoy!

39. Cherry tomatoes with mozzarella balls

Ingredient:

- 1 pint cherry or grape tomatoes, halved
- 8 oz fresh mozzarella balls, halved
- 2 tbsp extra virgin olive oil
- 1 tbsp balsamic vinegar
- 1 tsp dried oregano
- 1/4 tsp salt
- 1/4 tsp black pepper
- 2 tbsp fresh basil leaves, chopped

Instructions:

1. In a medium bowl, combine the halved cherry tomatoes and mozzarella balls.

2. Drizzle the olive oil and balsamic vinegar over the tomatoes and mozzarella. Sprinkle with the oregano, salt, and black pepper. Gently toss to coat.

3. Top with the chopped fresh basil leaves.

4. Serve immediately or refrigerate until ready to serve.

This dish is great for both weight loss and muscle gain for a few reasons:

Weight Loss:
- The tomatoes and mozzarella provide protein, fiber, and healthy fats to keep you feeling full.
- The portion size is controlled, making it easy to incorporate into a calorie•controlled diet.
- The olive oil and balsamic vinegar add flavor without a lot of extra calories.

Muscle Gain:
- The mozzarella cheese is a good source of high•quality protein to support muscle building.
- The healthy fats from the olive oil help with nutrient absorption and hormone production.
- The dish is easy to prepare and portable, making it a convenient snack or side dish.

This simple, flavorful salad is a great way to get in some nutritious veggies, protein, and healthy fats. Enjoy!

40. Rice cakes with avocado

Ingredient:

- 2 whole grain rice cakes
- 1/2 ripe avocado, mashed
- 1 tbsp lemon juice
- 1/4 tsp salt
- 1/8 tsp black pepper
- 1 tbsp chopped fresh cilantro (optional)

Instructions:

1. In a small bowl, mash the avocado with a fork. Stir in the lemon juice, salt, and black pepper until well combined.

2. Spread the avocado mixture evenly over the two rice cakes.

3. Top with the chopped cilantro, if using.

This snack is great for both weight loss and muscle gain for the following reasons:

Weight Loss:
- The rice cakes provide complex carbs and fiber to help keep you feeling full.
- Avocado is a source of healthy monounsaturated fats, which can help promote feelings of satiety.
- The portion size is controlled, making it easy to incorporate into a calorie•controlled diet.

Muscle Gain:
- The avocado provides healthy fats that support hormone production and nutrient absorption, which is important for building muscle.
- The rice cakes provide carbohydrates to fuel your workouts and replenish glycogen stores.
- This snack is easy to prepare and portable, making it a convenient option before or after exercise.

Overall, this simple rice cake and avocado combo provides a nutritious balance of complex carbs, healthy fats, and a touch of protein to support both weight loss and muscle gain goals. Enjoy!

41. Baked chicken breast with quinoa and steamed broccoli

Ingredient:

- 4 boneless, skinless chicken breasts (about 6 oz each)
- 1 cup uncooked quinoa, rinsed
- 2 cups low•sodium chicken broth
- 1 lb broccoli florets
- 1 tbsp olive oil
- 1 tsp garlic powder
- 1 tsp dried oregano
- 1/2 tsp salt
- 1/4 tsp black pepper

Instructions:

1. Preheat oven to 400°F. Line a baking sheet with parchment paper.

2. Place the chicken breasts on the prepared baking sheet. Drizzle with 1 tsp of the olive oil and season with the garlic powder, oregano, salt, and pepper. Bake for 25•30 minutes, until the chicken is cooked through.

3. While the chicken is baking, prepare the quinoa. In a medium saucepan, combine the quinoa and chicken broth. Bring to a boil, then reduce heat to low, cover, and simmer for 15•20 minutes, until the quinoa is tender and the liquid is absorbed.

4. In a steamer basket, steam the broccoli florets for 5•7 minutes, until tender•crisp. Serve the baked chicken breast over the cooked quinoa, with the steamed broccoli on the side.

This meal is great for both weight loss and muscle gain for the following reasons:

Weight Loss:
- The chicken breast and quinoa provide lean protein to help keep you feeling full.
- The broccoli is low in calories but high in fiber, vitamins, and minerals.
- The portion sizes are balanced and controlled, making it easy to incorporate into a calorie•controlled diet.

Muscle Gain:
- The chicken breast is an excellent source of high•quality protein to support muscle building and repair.
- The quinoa provides complex carbohydrates to fuel your workouts and replenish glycogen stores.
- The healthy fats from the olive oil help with nutrient absorption and hormone production.

42. Grilled shrimp skewers with bell peppers and onions

Ingredient:

- 1 lb large shrimp, peeled and deveined
- 1 red bell pepper, cut into 1•inch pieces
- 1 yellow bell pepper, cut into 1•inch pieces
- 1 red onion, cut into 1•inch pieces
- 2 tbsp olive oil
- 1 tbsp lemon juice
- 1 tsp garlic powder
- 1 tsp dried oregano
- 1/2 tsp salt
- 1/4 tsp black pepper

Instructions:

1. In a large bowl, combine the shrimp, bell pepper pieces, and onion pieces.

2. In a small bowl, whisk together the olive oil, lemon juice, garlic powder, oregano, salt, and black pepper.

3. Pour the marinade over the shrimp and vegetables and toss to coat evenly.

4. Thread the shrimp, bell peppers, and onions onto metal or wooden skewers, alternating the ingredients.

5. Preheat grill or grill pan to medium•high heat.

6. Grill the skewers for 2•3 minutes per side, or until the shrimp are opaque and cooked through. Serve the grilled shrimp skewers immediately.

This dish is great for both weight loss and muscle gain for the following reasons:

Weight Loss:
- Shrimp is a lean protein that helps keep you feeling full without a lot of calories.
- The bell peppers and onions are low in calories but high in fiber, vitamins, and minerals.
- The portion sizes are controlled, making it easy to incorporate into a calorie•controlled diet.

This flavorful and nutritious grilled shrimp skewer dish is a great option for both weight loss and muscle gain. Enjoy!

43. Turkey burger with sweet potato fries

Ingredient:

Turkey Burgers:
• 1 lb ground turkey
• 1 tsp garlic powder
• 1 tsp onion powder
• 1/2 tsp salt
• 1/4 tsp black pepper
• 4 whole wheat burger buns

Sweet Potato Fries:
• 2 medium sweet potatoes, peeled and cut into 1/2•inch thick fries
• 1 tbsp olive oil
• 1/2 tsp paprika
• 1/4 tsp salt

Instructions:

Sweet Potato Fries:
1. Preheat oven to 400°F. Line a baking sheet with parchment paper.

2. In a large bowl, toss the sweet potato fries with the olive oil, paprika, and salt until evenly coated.

3. Spread the fries in a single layer on the prepared baking sheet. Bake for 20•25 minutes, flipping halfway, until crispy.

Turkey Burgers:
1. In a medium bowl, combine the ground turkey, garlic powder, onion powder, salt, and pepper. Mix well.

2. Form the mixture into 4 equal•sized patties.

3. Grill or cook the patties in a skillet over medium heat for 4•5 minutes per side, until cooked through. Serve the turkey burgers on the whole wheat buns with your desired toppings.

This well•rounded meal of a turkey burger and sweet potato fries is a delicious and nutritious option to support both your weight loss and muscle gain goals.

44. Stuffed portobello mushrooms with quinoa and spinach

Ingredient:

- 4 large portobello mushroom caps, stems removed and chopped
- 1 cup cooked quinoa
- 1 cup fresh spinach, chopped
- 1/4 cup crumbled feta cheese
- 2 tbsp olive oil
- 2 cloves garlic, minced
- 1/4 tsp salt
- 1/8 tsp black pepper

Instructions:

1. Preheat oven to 400°F. Line a baking sheet with parchment paper.

2. In a medium bowl, combine the chopped mushroom stems, cooked quinoa, spinach, feta cheese, 1 tbsp of the olive oil, garlic, salt, and pepper. Mix well.

3. Brush the portobello mushroom caps with the remaining 1 tbsp of olive oil and place them cap•side down on the prepared baking sheet.

4. Divide the quinoa•spinach mixture evenly among the mushroom caps, packing it in gently.

5. Bake for 15•20 minutes, until the mushrooms are tender and the filling is hot. Serve the stuffed portobello mushrooms immediately.

This dish is great for both weight loss and muscle gain for the following reasons:

Weight Loss:

- Portobello mushrooms are low in calories but high in fiber and nutrients.
- Quinoa is a high•protein, high•fiber grain that helps keep you feeling full.
- Spinach is low in calories but packed with vitamins, minerals, and antioxidants.
- The portion sizes are controlled, making it easy to incorporate into a calorie•controlled diet.

Muscle Gain:

- The quinoa provides complex carbohydrates to fuel your workouts and replenish glycogen stores.
- The feta cheese adds a boost of protein to support muscle building and repair.
- The healthy fats from the olive oil help with nutrient absorption and hormone production

45. Salmon salad with avocado and mixed greens

Ingredient:

- 4 oz cooked salmon fillet, flaked
- 1/2 avocado, diced
- 2 cups mixed greens (such as spinach, arugula, and kale)
- 1 tbsp olive oil
- 1 tbsp lemon juice
- 1 tsp Dijon mustard
- 1/4 tsp salt
- 1/8 tsp black pepper

Instructions:

1. In a medium bowl, gently toss the flaked salmon and diced avocado.

2. In a small bowl, whisk together the olive oil, lemon juice, Dijon mustard, salt, and black pepper to make the dressing.

3. Add the mixed greens to the salmon and avocado, then drizzle the dressing over the top. Toss gently to coat.

4. Serve the salmon salad immediately.

This dish is great for both weight loss and muscle gain for the following reasons:

Weight Loss:
- Salmon is a lean protein that helps keep you feeling full without a lot of calories.
- Avocado provides healthy fats that can help promote feelings of satiety.
- The mixed greens are low in calories but high in fiber, vitamins, and minerals.
- The portion sizes are controlled, making it easy to incorporate into a calorie•controlled diet.

Muscle Gain:
- Salmon is an excellent source of high•quality protein to support muscle building and repair.
- The healthy fats from the avocado and olive oil help with nutrient absorption and hormone production.
- The greens provide complex carbohydrates to fuel your workouts and replenish glycogen stores.

46. Zucchini noodles with pesto and grilled chicken

Ingredient:

- 2 medium zucchinis, spiralized or julienned into noodles
- 1/4 cup basil pesto (store•bought or homemade)
- 1 lb boneless, skinless chicken breasts
- 1 tbsp olive oil
- 1 tsp garlic powder
- 1/2 tsp salt
- 1/4 tsp black pepper

Instructions:

1. Preheat grill or grill pan to medium•high heat.

2. Season the chicken breasts with the garlic powder, salt, and pepper.

3. Grill the chicken for 5•7 minutes per side, until cooked through. Allow to rest for 5 minutes, then slice or shred the chicken.

4. In a large bowl, toss the zucchini noodles with the basil pesto until evenly coated.

5. Divide the pesto zucchini noodles into serving bowls and top with the grilled chicken.

This dish is great for both weight loss and muscle gain for the following reasons:

Weight Loss:
- Zucchini noodles are a low•calorie, high•fiber alternative to traditional pasta.
- Chicken breast is a lean protein that helps keep you feeling full without a lot of calories.
- The portion sizes are controlled, making it easy to incorporate into a calorie•controlled diet.

Muscle Gain:
- The chicken breast provides high•quality protein to support muscle building and repair.
- The healthy fats from the olive oil and pesto help with nutrient absorption and hormone production.
- The zucchini noodles offer complex carbohydrates to fuel your workouts and replenish glycogen stores.

47. Baked tilapia with brown rice and green beans

Ingredient:

- 4 tilapia fillets (about 4-6 oz each)
- 1 tbsp olive oil
- 1 tsp lemon juice
- 1 tsp garlic powder
- 1/2 tsp paprika
- 1/4 tsp salt
- 1/8 tsp black pepper
- 1 cup uncooked brown rice
- 1 lb fresh green beans, trimmed
- 1 tbsp water

Instructions:

1. Preheat oven to 400°F. Line a baking sheet with parchment paper.

2. In a small bowl, mix together the olive oil, lemon juice, garlic powder, paprika, salt, and pepper. Brush the mixture evenly over the tilapia fillets.

3. Place the tilapia on the prepared baking sheet and bake for 15-18 minutes, until the fish flakes easily with a fork.

4. While the fish is baking, cook the brown rice according to package instructions.

5. In a steamer basket, steam the green beans with the 1 tbsp of water for 5-7 minutes, until tender-crisp.

6. Serve the baked tilapia over the cooked brown rice, with the steamed green beans on the side.

This meal is great for both weight loss and muscle gain for the following reasons:

Weight Loss:
- Tilapia is a lean, low-calorie protein that helps keep you feeling full.
- Brown rice is a complex carbohydrate that provides sustained energy without a lot of calories.
- Green beans are low in calories but high in fiber, vitamins, and minerals.
- The portion sizes are balanced and controlled, making it easy to incorporate into a calorie-controlled diet

48. Chicken and avocado Caesar salad

Ingredient:

- 4 cups chopped romaine lettuce
- 1 grilled or baked chicken breast, sliced
- 1/2 avocado, diced
- 2 tbsp grated Parmesan cheese
- 2 tbsp Caesar dressing (use a low·calorie or homemade version)
- 1 tbsp toasted whole wheat croutons (optional)
- 1/4 tsp black pepper

Instructions:

1. In a large salad bowl, combine the chopped romaine lettuce, sliced chicken breast, and diced avocado.

2. Drizzle the Caesar dressing over the salad and toss gently to coat.

3. Sprinkle the Parmesan cheese and black pepper over the top. If desired, top with a few toasted whole wheat croutons. Serve immediately.

This salad is great for both weight loss and muscle gain for the following reasons:

Weight Loss:
- Romaine lettuce is low in calories but high in fiber, vitamins, and minerals.
- Chicken breast is a lean protein that helps keep you feeling full without a lot of calories.
- Avocado provides healthy fats that can help promote feelings of satiety.
- The portion sizes are controlled, making it easy to incorporate into a calorie·controlled diet.

Muscle Gain:
- The chicken breast provides high·quality protein to support muscle building and repair.
- The healthy fats from the avocado help with nutrient absorption and hormone production.
- The Parmesan cheese adds a boost of protein to the meal.

This flavorful and nutrient·dense chicken and avocado Caesar salad is a great option for both weight loss and muscle gain. The combination of lean protein, healthy fats, and fiber·rich greens makes it a well·balanced and satisfying meal.

49. Beef and broccoli stir·fry with brown rice

Ingredient:

- 1 lb flank steak, thinly sliced
- 3 cups broccoli florets
- 1 tbsp sesame oil
- 2 tbsp low·sodium soy sauce
- 1 tbsp rice vinegar
- 1 tsp honey
- 2 cloves garlic, minced
- 1/2 tsp ground ginger
- 1/4 tsp red pepper flakes (optional)
- 1 cup cooked brown rice

Instructions:

1. In a small bowl, whisk together the soy sauce, rice vinegar, honey, garlic, ginger, and red pepper flakes (if using). Set aside.

2. Heat the sesame oil in a large skillet or wok over high heat. Add the sliced beef and stir·fry for 2·3 minutes, until browned.

3. Add the broccoli florets to the skillet and continue to stir·fry for 3·4 minutes, until the broccoli is tender·crisp.

4. Pour the soy sauce mixture into the skillet and toss everything together, cooking for an additional 1·2 minutes until the sauce has thickened slightly. Serve the beef and broccoli stir·fry over the cooked brown rice.

This dish is great for both weight loss and muscle gain for the following reasons:

Weight Loss:
- Flank steak is a lean protein that helps keep you feeling full without a lot of calories.
- Broccoli is low in calories but high in fiber, vitamins, and minerals.
- Brown rice is a complex carbohydrate that provides sustained energy without a lot of calories.
- The portion sizes are balanced and controlled, making it easy to incorporate into a calorie·controlled diet.

This flavorful and nutritious beef and broccoli stir·fry with brown rice is a great option to support both your weight loss and muscle gain goals. Enjoy!

50. Spinach and feta stuffed chicken breast

Ingredient:

- 4 boneless, skinless chicken breasts
- 1 cup fresh spinach, chopped
- 1/2 cup crumbled feta cheese
- 2 tbsp cream cheese, softened
- 1 clove garlic, minced
- 1/4 tsp dried oregano
- 1/4 tsp salt
- 1/8 tsp black pepper
- 1 tbsp olive oil

Instructions:

1. Preheat oven to 400°F. Line a baking sheet with parchment paper.

2. In a medium bowl, mix together the chopped spinach, feta cheese, cream cheese, garlic, oregano, salt, and pepper until well combined.

3. Use a sharp knife to cut a pocket into the side of each chicken breast, being careful not to cut all the way through.

4. Stuff each chicken breast with about 1/4 of the spinach and feta mixture, packing it in gently.

5. Place the stuffed chicken breasts on the prepared baking sheet. Drizzle the tops with the olive oil.

6. Bake for 25·30 minutes, until the chicken is cooked through and the internal temperature reaches 165°F. Serve the spinach and feta stuffed chicken breasts immediately.

This dish is a great option for both weight loss and muscle gain for the following reasons:

Weight Loss:
- Chicken breast is a lean protein that helps keep you feeling full without a lot of calories.
- Spinach is low in calories but high in fiber, vitamins, and minerals.
- The portion sizes are controlled, making it easy to incorporate into a calorie·controlled diet.

51. Turkey meatloaf with mashed cauliflower

Ingredient:

Turkey Meatloaf:
- 1 lb ground turkey
- 1/2 cup whole wheat breadcrumbs
- 1/4 cup diced onion
- 1 egg
- 2 tbsp ketchup
- 1 tsp Worcestershire sauce
- 1/2 tsp garlic powder
- 1/2 tsp dried oregano
- 1/4 tsp salt
- 1/4 tsp black pepper

Mashed Cauliflower:
- 1 head of cauliflower, cut into florets
- 2 tbsp unsweetened almond milk
- 1 tbsp grated Parmesan cheese
- 1/4 tsp salt
- 1/8 tsp black pepper

Instructions:

Turkey Meatloaf:
1. Preheat oven to 375°F. Lightly grease a 9x5 inch loaf pan.
2. In a large bowl, combine all the meatloaf ingredients and mix well.
3. Press the mixture into the prepared loaf pan.
4. Bake for 45•50 minutes, until the internal temperature reaches 165°F.
5. Let the meatloaf rest for 5 minutes before slicing.

Mashed Cauliflower:
1. In a large pot, bring water to a boil. Add the cauliflower florets and cook for 8•10 minutes, until very tender.
2. Drain the cauliflower and return it to the pot. Mash the cauliflower with a potato masher or hand mixer.
3. Stir in the almond milk, Parmesan cheese, salt, and pepper until well combined.

Serve the turkey meatloaf slices with the mashed cauliflower on the side.

This well•rounded meal of turkey meatloaf and mashed cauliflower is a delicious and nutritious option to support both your weight loss and muscle gain goals.

52. Grilled lamb chops with quinoa salad

Ingredient:

Lamb Chops:
• 4 lamb chops (about 4•6 oz each)
• 1 tbsp olive oil
• 1 tsp dried oregano
• 1/2 tsp garlic powder
• 1/4 tsp salt
• 1/8 tsp black pepper

Quinoa Salad:
• 1 cup cooked quinoa, cooled
• 1 cup diced cucumber
• 1/2 cup diced tomatoes
• 1/4 cup crumbled feta cheese
• 2 tbsp chopped fresh parsley
• 1 tbsp lemon juice
• 1 tbsp olive oil
• 1/4 tsp salt
• 1/8 tsp black pepper

Instructions:

1. Preheat grill or grill pan to medium•high heat.

2. In a small bowl, combine the olive oil, oregano, garlic powder, salt, and pepper. Rub the mixture evenly over the lamb chops.

3. Grill the lamb chops for 3•4 minutes per side, until they reach the desired doneness.

4. In a medium bowl, combine all the quinoa salad ingredients and toss gently to mix. Serve the grilled lamb chops with the quinoa salad on the side.

This meal is great for both weight loss and muscle gain for the following reasons:

Weight Loss:
• Lamb chops are a lean protein that helps keep you feeling full without a lot of calories.
• Quinoa is a high•protein, high•fiber grain that provides sustained energy.
• The vegetables in the quinoa salad are low in calories but high in fiber, vitamins, and minerals.
• The portion sizes are balanced and controlled, making it easy to incorporate into a calorie•controlled diet.

Muscle Gain:
• The lamb chops provide high•quality protein to support muscle building and repair.
• The healthy fats from the olive oil help with nutrient absorption and hormone production.
• The quinoa offers complex carbohydrates to fuel your workouts and replenish glycogen stores.
• The feta cheese adds a boost of protein to the salad

53. Shrimp and vegetable kebabs

Ingredient:

• 1 lb large shrimp, peeled and deveined
• 1 red bell pepper, cut into 1-inch pieces
• 1 yellow bell pepper, cut into 1-inch pieces
• 1 zucchini, cut into 1-inch pieces
• 1 red onion, cut into 1-inch pieces
• 2 tbsp olive oil
• 1 tbsp lemon juice
• 1 tsp garlic powder
• 1 tsp dried oregano
• 1/2 tsp salt
• 1/4 tsp black pepper

Instructions:

1. Preheat grill or grill pan to medium-high heat.

2. In a large bowl, combine the shrimp, bell pepper pieces, zucchini, and onion pieces.

3. In a small bowl, whisk together the olive oil, lemon juice, garlic powder, oregano, salt, and black pepper.

4. Pour the marinade over the shrimp and vegetables and toss to coat evenly.

5. Thread the shrimp and vegetables onto skewers, alternating the ingredients.

6. Grill the kebabs for 2-3 minutes per side, or until the shrimp are opaque and cooked through and the vegetables are tender. Serve the grilled shrimp and vegetable kebabs immediately.

This dish is great for both weight loss and muscle gain for the following reasons:

Weight Loss:
• Shrimp is a lean protein that helps keep you feeling full without a lot of calories.
• The vegetables (bell peppers, zucchini, onion) are low in calories but high in fiber, vitamins, and minerals.
• The portion sizes are controlled, making it easy to incorporate into a calorie-controlled diet.

This flavorful and nutritious grilled shrimp and vegetable kebab dish is a great option for both weight loss and muscle gain. The combination of lean protein, healthy fats, and fiber-rich vegetables makes it a well-balanced and satisfying meal.

54. Chicken and black bean burrito bowl

Ingredient:

- 1 lb boneless, skinless chicken breasts, grilled and shredded
- 1 (15 oz) can black beans, rinsed and drained
- 1 cup cooked brown rice
- 1 cup chopped romaine lettuce
- 1/2 cup diced tomatoes
- 1/4 cup diced red onion
- 2 tbsp shredded cheddar cheese
- 2 tbsp plain Greek yogurt
- 1 tbsp fresh cilantro, chopped
- 1 tbsp lime juice
- 1/2 tsp cumin
- 1/4 tsp chili powder
- 1/4 tsp salt
- 1/8 tsp black pepper

Instructions:

1. In a large bowl, combine the shredded chicken, black beans, brown rice, romaine lettuce, tomatoes, and red onion.

2. In a small bowl, mix together the Greek yogurt, cilantro, lime juice, cumin, chili powder, salt, and pepper.

3. Drizzle the yogurt dressing over the burrito bowl and toss gently to coat. Top the burrito bowl with the shredded cheddar cheese. Serve immediately.

This dish is great for both weight loss and muscle gain for the following reasons:

Weight Loss:
- Chicken breast is a lean protein that helps keep you feeling full without a lot of calories.
- Black beans are a good source of fiber and protein to aid in satiety.
- The vegetables (lettuce, tomatoes, onion) are low in calories but high in nutrients.
- The portion sizes are balanced and controlled, making it easy to incorporate into a calorie-controlled diet.

This flavorful and nutritious chicken and black bean burrito bowl is a great option to support both your weight loss and muscle gain goals. The combination of lean protein, complex carbs, and fiber-rich vegetables makes it a well-balanced and satisfying meal.

55. Roasted vegetable quinoa bowl

Ingredient:

- 1 cup uncooked quinoa, rinsed
- 2 cups low•sodium vegetable broth
- 1 medium zucchini, diced
- 1 red bell pepper, diced
- 1 cup broccoli florets
- 1 cup cherry tomatoes, halved
- 1 red onion, diced
- 2 tbsp olive oil
- 1 tsp dried oregano
- 1/2 tsp garlic powder
- 1/4 tsp salt
- 1/8 tsp black pepper
- 2 tbsp crumbled feta cheese (optional)
- 2 tbsp chopped fresh parsley

Instructions:

1. Preheat oven to 400°F. Line a large baking sheet with parchment paper.

2. In a large bowl, toss the diced zucchini, bell pepper, broccoli, tomatoes, and onion with the olive oil, oregano, garlic powder, salt, and pepper.

3. Spread the vegetables in a single layer on the prepared baking sheet. Roast for 20•25 minutes, stirring halfway, until the vegetables are tender and lightly browned.

4. While the vegetables are roasting, cook the quinoa according to package instructions using the vegetable broth.

5. Once the vegetables and quinoa are cooked, combine them in a large bowl. Stir in the feta cheese (if using) and chopped parsley. Serve the roasted vegetable quinoa bowl warm.

This flavorful and nutritious roasted vegetable quinoa bowl is a great option to support both your weight loss and muscle gain goals. The combination of complex carbs, lean protein, and fiber•rich vegetables makes it a well•balanced and satisfying meal.

56. Turkey and vegetable skewers

Ingredient:

- 1 lb ground turkey
- 1 red bell pepper, cut into 1·inch pieces
- 1 yellow bell pepper, cut into 1·inch pieces
- 1 zucchini, cut into 1·inch pieces
- 1 red onion, cut into 1·inch pieces
- 2 tbsp olive oil
- 1 tbsp lemon juice
- 1 tsp dried oregano
- 1/2 tsp garlic powder
- 1/2 tsp salt
- 1/4 tsp black pepper

Instructions:

1. Preheat grill or grill pan to medium·high heat.

2. In a large bowl, combine the ground turkey, bell pepper pieces, zucchini, and onion pieces. In a small bowl, whisk together the olive oil, lemon juice, oregano, garlic powder, salt, and black pepper.

3. Pour the marinade over the turkey and vegetables and toss to coat evenly. Thread the turkey mixture onto skewers, alternating the ingredients.

4. Grill the skewers for 8·10 minutes, turning occasionally, until the turkey is cooked through and the vegetables are tender. Serve the grilled turkey and vegetable skewers immediately.

This dish is great for both weight loss and muscle gain for the following reasons:
Muscle Gain:
- Ground turkey is an excellent source of high·quality protein to support muscle building and repair.
- The healthy fats from the olive oil help with nutrient absorption and hormone production.
- The grilled vegetables provide complex carbohydrates to fuel your workouts and replenish glycogen stores.

This flavorful and nutritious grilled turkey and vegetable skewer dish is a great option for both weight loss and muscle gain. The combination of lean protein, healthy fats, and fiber·rich vegetables makes it a well·balanced and satisfying meal.

57. Grilled chicken with avocado salsa

Ingredient:

Grilled Chicken:
- 4 boneless, skinless chicken breasts
- 1 tbsp olive oil
- 1 tsp chili powder
- 1/2 tsp garlic powder
- 1/4 tsp salt
- 1/8 tsp black pepper

Avocado Salsa:
- 1 ripe avocado, diced
- 1/2 cup diced tomatoes
- 2 tbsp diced red onion
- 1 tbsp chopped fresh cilantro
- 1 tbsp lime juice
- 1/4 tsp salt
- 1/8 tsp black pepper

Instructions:
1. Preheat grill or grill pan to medium·high heat.

2. In a small bowl, combine the olive oil, chili powder, garlic powder, salt, and pepper. Rub the mixture evenly over the chicken breasts.

3. Grill the chicken for 5·7 minutes per side, until cooked through and no longer pink in the center.

4. In a medium bowl, gently mix together all the avocado salsa ingredients. Serve the grilled chicken topped with the avocado salsa.

This dish is great for both weight loss and muscle gain for the following reasons:
Muscle Gain:
- The chicken breast provides high·quality protein to support muscle building and repair.
- The healthy fats from the avocado and olive oil help with nutrient absorption and hormone production.
- The salsa offers a flavorful way to add more vegetables to the meal.

This grilled chicken with avocado salsa is a delicious and nutritious option that can support both your weight loss and muscle gain goals. The combination of lean protein, healthy fats, and fiber·rich vegetables makes it a well·balanced and satisfying meal.

58. Lentil and vegetable curry

Ingredient:

- 1 cup dry brown lentils, rinsed
- 2 cups low•sodium vegetable broth
- 1 tbsp olive oil
- 1 onion, diced
- 3 cloves garlic, minced
- 1 tbsp grated fresh ginger
- 2 tsp curry powder
- 1 tsp ground cumin
- 1/2 tsp ground turmeric
- 1/4 tsp cayenne pepper (optional)
- 1 cup diced tomatoes
- 1 cup diced cauliflower florets
- 1 cup diced sweet potato
- 1 cup chopped spinach
- 1/4 cup plain Greek yogurt
- 2 tbsp chopped fresh cilantro
- Salt and black pepper to taste

Instructions:

1. In a medium saucepan, combine the lentils and vegetable broth. Bring to a boil, then reduce heat and simmer for 15•20 minutes, until lentils are tender.

2. In a large skillet, heat the olive oil over medium heat. Add the onion and sauté for 3•4 minutes until translucent.

3. Add the garlic, ginger, curry powder, cumin, turmeric, and cayenne (if using). Cook for 1 minute, stirring constantly, until fragrant.

4. Stir in the diced tomatoes, cauliflower, and sweet potato. Simmer for 10•12 minutes, until vegetables are tender.

5. Add the cooked lentils and spinach to the skillet. Cook for 2•3 minutes, until the spinach is wilted.

6. Remove from heat and stir in the Greek yogurt and chopped cilantro. Season with salt and black pepper to taste. Serve the lentil and vegetable curry warm.

59. Shrimp and avocado salad

Ingredient:

- 1 lb cooked shrimp, peeled and deveined
- 1 ripe avocado, diced
- 1 cup cherry tomatoes, halved
- 1/2 cup diced cucumber
- 1/4 cup diced red onion
- 2 tbsp chopped fresh cilantro
- 2 tbsp lime juice
- 1 tbsp olive oil
- 1/4 tsp salt
- 1/8 tsp black pepper

Instructions:

1. In a large bowl, combine the cooked shrimp, diced avocado, cherry tomatoes, cucumber, red onion, and chopped cilantro.

2. In a small bowl, whisk together the lime juice, olive oil, salt, and black pepper to make the dressing.

3. Pour the dressing over the shrimp and avocado salad and toss gently to coat. Serve the shrimp and avocado salad immediately.

This salad is great for both weight loss and muscle gain for the following reasons:
Weight Loss:
- Shrimp is a lean protein that helps keep you feeling full without a lot of calories.
- Avocado provides healthy fats that can help promote feelings of satiety.
- The vegetables (tomatoes, cucumber, onion) are low in calories but high in fiber, vitamins, and minerals.
- The portion sizes are controlled, making it easy to incorporate into a calorie·controlled diet.

Muscle Gain:
- Shrimp is an excellent source of high·quality protein to support muscle building and repair.
- The healthy fats from the avocado and olive oil help with nutrient absorption and hormone production.
- The salad provides a nutrient·dense way to get in a variety of vegetables

60. Beef stir·fry with mixed vegetables

Ingredient:

- 1 lb flank steak, thinly sliced
- 2 tbsp low·sodium soy sauce
- 1 tbsp rice vinegar
- 1 tsp sesame oil
- 1 tsp honey
- 2 cloves garlic, minced
- 1 tbsp olive oil
- 1 cup broccoli florets
- 1 cup sliced mushrooms
- 1 red bell pepper, sliced
- 1 cup snow peas
- 1/2 cup sliced water chestnuts
- 2 cups cooked brown rice

Instructions:

1. In a small bowl, whisk together the soy sauce, rice vinegar, sesame oil, honey, and garlic. Set aside.

2. Heat the olive oil in a large skillet or wok over high heat. Add the sliced beef and stir·fry for 2·3 minutes, until browned.

3. Add the broccoli, mushrooms, bell pepper, snow peas, and water chestnuts to the skillet. Stir·fry for 4·5 minutes, until the vegetables are tender·crisp.

4. Pour the soy sauce mixture into the skillet and toss everything together, cooking for an additional 1·2 minutes until the sauce has thickened slightly. Serve the beef and vegetable stir·fry over the cooked brown rice.

This dish is great for both weight loss and muscle gain for the following reasons:

Weight Loss:
- Flank steak is a lean protein that helps keep you feeling full without a lot of calories.
- The mixed vegetables (broccoli, mushrooms, bell pepper, snow peas) are low in calories but high in fiber, vitamins, and minerals.
- Brown rice is a complex carbohydrate that provides sustained energy without a lot of calories.
- The portion sizes are balanced and controlled, making it easy to incorporate into a calorie·controlled diet

61. Chicken and sweet potato skillet

Ingredient:

- 1 lb boneless, skinless chicken breasts, cubed
- 2 medium sweet potatoes, peeled and cubed
- 1 onion, diced
- 2 cloves garlic, minced
- 1 tsp paprika
- 1 tsp dried thyme
- Salt and pepper to taste
- 1 tbsp olive oil

Instructions:

1. Heat the olive oil in a large skillet over medium·high heat.

2. Add the cubed chicken and cook for 5·7 minutes, stirring occasionally, until the chicken is lightly browned.

3. Add the diced onion and minced garlic. Cook for 2·3 minutes until the onion is translucent.

4. Add the cubed sweet potatoes, paprika, thyme, salt, and pepper. Stir to combine.

5. Cover the skillet and cook for 15·20 minutes, stirring occasionally, until the sweet potatoes are tender.

6. Remove the lid and continue cooking for 5 more minutes to allow the flavors to meld.

7. Serve hot.

This dish is high in protein from the chicken, and the sweet potatoes provide complex carbs, fiber, and nutrients. It's a balanced meal that can support both weight loss and muscle gain when paired with a healthy overall diet and exercise routine.

62. Baked salmon with dill yogurt sauce

Ingredient:

• 4 (6 oz) salmon fillets
• 1 tbsp olive oil
• Salt and pepper to taste

For the Dill Yogurt Sauce:
• 1 cup plain Greek yogurt
• 2 tbsp fresh dill, chopped
• 1 tbsp lemon juice
• 1 garlic clove, minced
• Salt and pepper to taste

Instructions:

1. Preheat the oven to 400°F.

2. Place the salmon fillets on a baking sheet lined with parchment paper. Drizzle with olive oil and season with salt and pepper.

3. Bake the salmon for 12•15 minutes, or until it flakes easily with a fork.

4. While the salmon is baking, make the dill yogurt sauce. In a small bowl, mix together the Greek yogurt, fresh dill, lemon juice, garlic, salt, and pepper.

5. Serve the baked salmon warm, topped with the dill yogurt sauce.

This dish is high in protein from the salmon, and the yogurt sauce provides a creamy, tangy flavor. The healthy fats from the salmon and the nutrients from the dill and yogurt make this a great option for both weight loss and muscle gain when paired with a balanced diet and exercise routine.

63. Turkey and spinach stuffed mushrooms

Ingredient:

- 12 large mushrooms, stems removed and finely chopped
- 1 lb ground turkey
- 1 cup fresh spinach, chopped
- 2 cloves garlic, minced
- 1/4 cup grated Parmesan cheese
- 2 tbsp breadcrumbs
- 1 tbsp olive oil
- Salt and pepper to taste

Instructions:

1. Preheat the oven to 375°F.

2. In a skillet, cook the ground turkey over medium heat until no longer pink, 5-7 minutes. Drain any excess fat.

3. Add the chopped mushroom stems, spinach, and garlic to the skillet. Cook for 2-3 minutes until the spinach is wilted.

4. Remove the skillet from heat and stir in the Parmesan cheese and breadcrumbs. Season with salt and pepper.

5. Arrange the mushroom caps on a baking sheet. Spoon the turkey and spinach mixture into the mushroom caps.

6. Bake for 12-15 minutes, or until the mushrooms are tender and the filling is hot.

7. Serve warm.

These stuffed mushrooms are a great source of protein from the ground turkey, and the spinach provides fiber and nutrients. The Parmesan cheese and breadcrumbs add a nice texture and flavor. This dish can be a healthy appetizer or side dish that supports both weight loss and muscle gain when part of a balanced diet and exercise routine.

64. Shrimp and asparagus stir·fry

Ingredient:

- 1 lb shrimp, peeled and deveined
- 1 lb asparagus, trimmed and cut into 1·inch pieces
- 2 tbsp olive oil
- 3 cloves garlic, minced
- 1 tbsp grated ginger
- 2 tbsp low·sodium soy sauce
- 1 tbsp rice vinegar
- 1 tsp sesame oil
- Salt and pepper to taste
- Chopped green onions for garnish (optional)

Instructions:

1. Heat the olive oil in a large skillet or wok over high heat.

2. Add the shrimp and stir·fry for 2·3 minutes until they start to turn pink.

3. Add the asparagus, garlic, and ginger. Stir·fry for 3·4 minutes until the asparagus is tender·crisp.

4. In a small bowl, whisk together the soy sauce, rice vinegar, and sesame oil.

5. Pour the sauce into the skillet and toss everything together until the shrimp is cooked through and the sauce has thickened slightly, about 2 minutes.

6. Season with salt and pepper to taste.

7. Serve immediately, garnished with chopped green onions if desired.

This stir·fry is high in protein from the shrimp and low in carbs, making it a great option for both weight loss and muscle gain. The asparagus provides fiber, vitamins, and minerals. Pair this dish with a side of brown rice or quinoa for a complete, balanced meal.

65. Grilled vegetable and quinoa salad

Ingredient:

- 1 cup uncooked quinoa, rinsed
- 2 cups vegetable or chicken broth
- 1 zucchini, sliced
- 1 yellow squash, sliced
- 1 red bell pepper, sliced
- 1 red onion, sliced
- 2 tbsp olive oil
- Salt and pepper to taste
- 1/4 cup crumbled feta cheese (optional)
- 2 tbsp chopped fresh parsley

For the Dressing:
- 2 tbsp olive oil
- 2 tbsp balsamic vinegar
- 1 tbsp Dijon mustard
- 1 clove garlic, minced
- Salt and pepper to taste

Instructions:

1. Cook the quinoa according to package instructions using the broth instead of water. Fluff with a fork and set aside to cool.

2. Preheat grill or grill pan to medium•high heat.

3. Toss the sliced vegetables with 2 tbsp of olive oil and season with salt and pepper.

4. Grill the vegetables for 5•7 minutes per side, or until tender and slightly charred.

5. In a large bowl, combine the cooked quinoa, grilled vegetables, feta cheese (if using), and parsley.

6. In a small bowl, whisk together the dressing ingredients. Pour the dressing over the quinoa salad and toss to coat. Serve chilled or at room temperature.

This salad is packed with fiber, protein, and nutrients from the quinoa, grilled vegetables, and optional feta cheese. The dressing adds a flavorful touch. This dish can be a great option for both weight loss and muscle gain when part of a balanced diet and exercise routine.

66. Chicken and chickpea salad

Ingredient:

- 2 cups cooked, shredded chicken breast
- 1 (15 oz) can chickpeas, drained and rinsed
- 1 cup diced cucumber
- 1/2 cup diced red onion
- 1/2 cup diced bell pepper
- 2 tbsp chopped fresh parsley
- 2 tbsp olive oil
- 2 tbsp lemon juice
- 1 tsp Dijon mustard
- Salt and pepper to taste

Instructions:

1. In a large bowl, combine the shredded chicken, chickpeas, cucumber, red onion, bell pepper, and parsley.

2. In a small bowl, whisk together the olive oil, lemon juice, and Dijon mustard. Season with salt and pepper.

3. Pour the dressing over the chicken and chickpea mixture and toss to coat everything evenly.

4. Refrigerate the salad for at least 30 minutes to allow the flavors to meld.

5. Serve chilled or at room temperature.

This salad is a great source of protein from the chicken and fiber from the chickpeas. The vegetables add crunch and nutrients. The simple dressing adds flavor without adding a lot of extra calories or fat.

This dish can be a great option for both weight loss and muscle gain when paired with a balanced diet and exercise routine. The protein and fiber will help keep you feeling full and satisfied, while the nutrient•dense ingredients support overall health and fitness goals.

67. Beef and vegetable kebabs

Ingredient:

- 1 lb beef sirloin or tenderloin, cut into 1·inch cubes
- 1 red bell pepper, cut into 1·inch pieces
- 1 yellow bell pepper, cut into 1·inch pieces
- 1 red onion, cut into 1·inch pieces
- 8 oz mushrooms, halved
- 2 tbsp olive oil
- 2 tbsp balsamic vinegar
- 1 tsp dried oregano
- 1 tsp garlic powder
- Salt and pepper to taste

Instructions:

1. In a large bowl, combine the beef cubes, bell pepper pieces, onion pieces, and mushrooms.

2. In a small bowl, whisk together the olive oil, balsamic vinegar, oregano, garlic powder, salt, and pepper.

3. Pour the marinade over the beef and vegetables and toss to coat everything evenly.

4. Thread the marinated beef and vegetables onto skewers, alternating the ingredients.

5. Preheat grill or grill pan to medium·high heat.

6. Grill the kebabs for 10·12 minutes, turning occasionally, until the beef is cooked through and the vegetables are tender. Serve the beef and vegetable kebabs immediately.

These kebabs are a great source of lean protein from the beef, and the vegetables provide fiber, vitamins, and minerals. The marinade adds flavor without a lot of extra calories or fat.

This dish can be a great option for both weight loss and muscle gain when paired with a balanced diet and exercise routine. The protein from the beef supports muscle growth and maintenance, while the vegetables and lean meat help with weight management.

68. Grilled fish tacos with avocado salsa

Ingredient:

For the Fish:
- 1 lb white fish fillets
(such as tilapia, cod, or halibut)
- 1 tbsp olive oil
- 1 tsp chili powder
- 1 tsp cumin
- Salt and pepper to taste

For Serving:
- 8-10 small corn or flour tortillas
- Shredded cabbage or lettuce
- Lime wedges

For the Avocado Salsa:
- 2 avocados, diced
- 1 tomato, diced
- 1/4 cup diced red onion
- 2 tbsp chopped cilantro
- 1 tbsp lime juice
- Salt and pepper to taste

Instructions:

1. Preheat grill or grill pan to medium·high heat.

2. In a shallow dish, rub the fish fillets with olive oil and season with chili powder, cumin, salt, and pepper.

3. Grill the fish for 3·4 minutes per side, or until it flakes easily with a fork.

4. In a medium bowl, combine the diced avocado, tomato, red onion, cilantro, and lime juice. Season with salt and pepper.

5. Warm the tortillas according to package instructions.

6. To assemble the tacos, place a piece of grilled fish in each tortilla, top with shredded cabbage or lettuce, and spoon the avocado salsa over the top.

7. Serve immediately with lime wedges.

These fish tacos are a great source of lean protein from the grilled fish, and the avocado salsa provides healthy fats, fiber, and nutrients. The combination of lean protein, healthy fats, and complex carbs from the tortillas makes this a well·balanced meal that can support both weight loss and muscle gain when part of a healthy diet and exercise routine.

69. Turkey and quinoa stuffed bell peppers

Ingredient:

- 4 bell peppers, halved and seeded
- 1 lb ground turkey
- 1 cup cooked quinoa
- 1 small onion, diced
- 2 cloves garlic, minced
- 1 (14.5 oz) can diced tomatoes
- 1 tsp dried oregano
- 1 tsp chili powder
- Salt and pepper to taste
- 1/2 cup shredded mozzarella cheese (optional)

Instructions:

1. Preheat the oven to 375°F.

2. In a large skillet, cook the ground turkey over medium heat until no longer pink, 5•7 minutes. Drain any excess fat.

3. Add the diced onion and minced garlic to the skillet. Cook for 2•3 minutes until the onion is translucent.

4. Stir in the cooked quinoa, diced tomatoes, oregano, chili powder, salt, and pepper. Cook for an additional 5 minutes.

5. Arrange the bell pepper halves in a baking dish. Spoon the turkey and quinoa mixture into the pepper halves.

6. If using, sprinkle the shredded mozzarella cheese over the top of the stuffed peppers.

7. Bake for 20•25 minutes, or until the peppers are tender and the filling is hot. Serve the stuffed peppers warm.

These stuffed bell peppers are a great source of lean protein from the ground turkey, complex carbs from the quinoa, and fiber and nutrients from the bell peppers. The optional mozzarella cheese adds a creamy texture.

This dish can be a great option for both weight loss and muscle gain when part of a balanced diet and exercise routine. The combination of macronutrients supports satiety and muscle growth.

70. Chicken and vegetable curry

Ingredient:

- 1 lb boneless,
skinless chicken breasts, cubed
- 2 tbsp olive oil
- 1 onion, diced
- 3 cloves garlic, minced
- 1 tbsp grated ginger
- 2 tsp curry powder
- 1 tsp ground cumin
- 1 tsp ground coriander
- 1 cup low•sodium chicken broth
- 1 (14 oz) can diced tomatoes
- 1 cup cauliflower florets
- 1 cup broccoli florets
- 1 cup diced sweet potato
- 1/2 cup frozen peas
- 1 tsp turmeric
- 1/4 cup plain Greek yogurt
- Salt and pepper to taste
- Chopped cilantro for garnish (optional)

Instructions:

1. In a large skillet or Dutch oven, heat the olive oil over medium•high heat.

2. Add the cubed chicken and cook for 5•7 minutes, until lightly browned. Remove the chicken from the skillet and set aside.

3. Add the diced onion, minced garlic, and grated ginger to the skillet. Cook for 2•3 minutes until the onion is translucent.

4. Stir in the curry powder, cumin, coriander, and turmeric. Cook for 1 minute to toast the spices.

5. Pour in the chicken broth and diced tomatoes. Bring the mixture to a simmer.

6. Add the cauliflower, broccoli, sweet potato, and peas to the skillet. Reduce heat to medium•low and simmer for 15•20 minutes, until the vegetables are tender.

7. Return the cooked chicken to the skillet and stir in the Greek yogurt. Season with salt and pepper to taste.

8. Serve the chicken and vegetable curry over steamed basmati rice, garnished with chopped cilantro if desired.

This curry dish is packed with lean protein from the chicken, complex carbs from the vegetables, and healthy fats from the olive oil and yogurt. The blend of spices adds flavor without a lot of extra calories or sodium.

This recipe can be a great option for both weight loss and muscle gain when incorporated into a balanced diet and exercise routine.

71. Salmon and avocado bowl

Ingredient:

- 4 (6 oz) salmon fillets
- 2 tbsp olive oil
- Salt and pepper to taste
- 2 cups cooked quinoa
- 1 avocado, diced
- 1 cup cherry tomatoes, halved
- 1/2 cup diced cucumber
- 2 tbsp chopped fresh cilantro
- 2 tbsp fresh lemon juice
- 1 tbsp olive oil
- Salt and pepper to taste

Instructions:

1. Preheat the oven to 400°F.

2. Place the salmon fillets on a baking sheet lined with parchment paper. Drizzle with 2 tbsp of olive oil and season with salt and pepper.

3. Bake the salmon for 12•15 minutes, or until it flakes easily with a fork.

4. In a large bowl, combine the cooked quinoa, diced avocado, cherry tomatoes, diced cucumber, and chopped cilantro.

5. In a small bowl, whisk together the lemon juice and 1 tbsp of olive oil. Season with salt and pepper. Pour the dressing over the quinoa and vegetable mixture and toss to coat.

6. Divide the quinoa salad evenly among 4 bowls. Top each bowl with a baked salmon fillet. Serve immediately.

This salmon and avocado bowl is a nutrient•dense meal that's great for both weight loss and muscle gain. The salmon provides lean protein and healthy omega•3 fatty acids, while the avocado, quinoa, and vegetables offer complex carbs, fiber, and a variety of vitamins and minerals.

The combination of protein, healthy fats, and complex carbs makes this dish a well•balanced option that can support your fitness goals when incorporated into an overall healthy diet and exercise routine.

72. Lentil and vegetable stew

Ingredient:

- 1 cup dry brown or green lentils, rinsed
- 4 cups low•sodium vegetable or chicken broth
- 1 tbsp olive oil
- 1 onion, diced
- 3 cloves garlic, minced
- 2 carrots, peeled and diced
- 2 celery stalks, diced
- 1 (14.5 oz) can diced tomatoes
- 2 cups chopped kale or spinach
- 1 tsp dried thyme
- 1 tsp dried oregano
- Salt and pepper to taste

Instructions:

1. In a large pot, combine the rinsed lentils and broth. Bring to a boil over high heat.

2. Reduce heat to medium•low, cover, and simmer for 15•20 minutes, or until the lentils are tender.

3. In a separate skillet, heat the olive oil over medium heat. Add the diced onion and sauté for 3•4 minutes until translucent.

4. Add the minced garlic, diced carrots, and diced celery to the skillet. Cook for an additional 5 minutes.

5. Transfer the sautéed vegetables to the pot with the cooked lentils. Add the diced tomatoes, chopped kale or spinach, thyme, and oregano.

6. Stir to combine and let the stew simmer for 10•15 minutes, until the vegetables are tender. Season with salt and pepper to taste. Serve the lentil and vegetable stew hot.

This hearty stew is packed with plant•based protein from the lentils, fiber and nutrients from the vegetables, and complex carbs. It's a well•balanced meal that can support both weight loss and muscle gain when incorporated into an overall healthy diet and exercise routine.

The lentils provide a good source of lean protein, while the vegetables and broth keep the dish low in calories and high in nutrients. This stew can be a satisfying and nutritious option for any fitness goal.

73. Chicken and broccoli stir•fry

Ingredient:

• 1 lb boneless, skinless chicken breasts, cut into 1•inch pieces
• 3 cups broccoli florets
• 2 tbsp low•sodium soy sauce
• 1 tbsp rice vinegar
• 1 tsp sesame oil
• 1 tsp cornstarch
• 2 tbsp olive oil
• 3 cloves garlic, minced
• 1 tbsp grated ginger
• Salt and pepper to taste
• Chopped green onions for garnish (optional)

Instructions:

1. In a small bowl, whisk together the soy sauce, rice vinegar, sesame oil, and cornstarch. Set aside.

2. Heat the olive oil in a large skillet or wok over high heat.

3. Add the chicken and stir•fry for 3•4 minutes until lightly browned.

4. Add the broccoli florets, minced garlic, and grated ginger. Stir•fry for an additional 3•4 minutes.

5. Pour the soy sauce mixture into the skillet and toss everything together. Cook for 2•3 minutes, or until the sauce has thickened and the chicken is cooked through.

6. Season with salt and pepper to taste. Serve the chicken and broccoli stir•fry immediately, garnished with chopped green onions if desired.

This stir•fry is a great option for both weight loss and muscle gain. The chicken provides lean protein to support muscle growth, while the broccoli is low in calories and high in fiber, vitamins, and minerals. The simple sauce adds flavor without a lot of extra calories or sodium.

Pair this dish with a side of steamed brown rice or quinoa for a complete, balanced meal that can support your fitness goals when incorporated into a healthy diet and exercise routine.

74. Turkey and vegetable chili

Ingredient:

- 1 lb ground turkey
- 1 onion, diced
- 3 cloves garlic, minced
- 1 red bell pepper, diced
- 1 zucchini, diced
- 1 (15 oz) can diced tomatoes
- 1 (15 oz) can kidney beans, drained and rinsed
- 1 (15 oz) can black beans, drained and rinsed
- 2 tbsp chili powder
- 1 tsp ground cumin
- 1 tsp dried oregano
- 1 tsp paprika
- Salt and pepper to taste
- Chopped cilantro for garnish (optional)

Instructions:

1. In a large pot or Dutch oven, cook the ground turkey over medium-high heat until browned and crumbled, 5-7 minutes. Drain any excess fat.

2. Add the diced onion and minced garlic to the pot. Cook for 2-3 minutes until the onion is translucent.

3. Stir in the diced red bell pepper and zucchini. Cook for an additional 5 minutes.

4. Pour in the diced tomatoes, kidney beans, and black beans. Add the chili powder, cumin, oregano, and paprika. Stir to combine.

5. Bring the chili to a simmer and let it cook for 20-25 minutes, stirring occasionally, until the vegetables are tender and the flavors have melded.

6. Season with salt and pepper to taste. Serve the turkey and vegetable chili hot, garnished with chopped cilantro if desired.

This chili is a great source of lean protein from the ground turkey, fiber and complex carbs from the beans and vegetables, and a variety of vitamins and minerals. The blend of spices adds flavor without a lot of extra calories or sodium.

This dish can be a great option for both weight loss and muscle gain when incorporated into a balanced diet and exercise routine. The combination of macronutrients and nutrients supports overall health and fitness goals.

75. Grilled chicken and vegetable kabobs

Ingredient:

- 1 lb boneless, skinless chicken breasts, cut into 1•inch cubes
- 1 red bell pepper, cut into 1•inch pieces
- 1 yellow bell pepper, cut into 1•inch pieces
- 1 zucchini, cut into 1•inch pieces
- 1 red onion, cut into 1•inch pieces
- 2 tbsp olive oil
- 2 tbsp lemon juice
- 1 tsp dried oregano
- 1 tsp garlic powder
- Salt and pepper to taste

Instructions:

1. In a large bowl, combine the cubed chicken, bell pepper pieces, zucchini pieces, and onion pieces.

2. In a small bowl, whisk together the olive oil, lemon juice, oregano, and garlic powder. Season with salt and pepper.

3. Pour the marinade over the chicken and vegetables and toss to coat everything evenly.

4. Thread the marinated chicken and vegetables onto skewers, alternating the ingredients.

5. Preheat grill or grill pan to medium•high heat.

6. Grill the kabobs for 12•15 minutes, turning occasionally, until the chicken is cooked through and the vegetables are tender. Serve the grilled chicken and vegetable kabobs immediately.

These kabobs are a great option for both weight loss and muscle gain. The chicken provides lean protein to support muscle growth, while the vegetables are low in calories and high in fiber, vitamins, and minerals.

The simple marinade adds flavor without a lot of extra calories or fat. Pair these kabobs with a side of quinoa or brown rice for a complete, balanced meal that can support your fitness goals when incorporated into a healthy diet and exercise routine.

76. Beef and cauliflower rice stir·fry

Ingredient:

- 1 lb lean beef sirloin, thinly sliced
- 2 tbsp low·sodium soy sauce
- 1 tbsp rice vinegar
- 1 tsp sesame oil
- 1 tsp cornstarch
- 2 tbsp olive oil

- 3 cloves garlic, minced
- 1 tbsp grated ginger
- 4 cups riced cauliflower
- 1 cup sliced mushrooms
- 1 cup diced bell pepper
- 2 green onions, sliced
- Salt and pepper to taste

Instructions:

1. In a small bowl, whisk together the soy sauce, rice vinegar, sesame oil, and cornstarch. Set aside.

2. Heat the olive oil in a large skillet or wok over high heat.

3. Add the sliced beef and stir·fry for 2·3 minutes until lightly browned.

4. Add the minced garlic and grated ginger to the skillet. Cook for 1 minute, stirring constantly.

5. Pour in the riced cauliflower, sliced mushrooms, and diced bell pepper. Stir·fry for 4·5 minutes until the vegetables are tender.

6. Pour the soy sauce mixture into the skillet and toss everything together. Cook for 2·3 minutes, or until the sauce has thickened.

7. Remove from heat and stir in the sliced green onions. Season with salt and pepper to taste. Serve the beef and cauliflower rice stir·fry immediately.

This stir·fry is a great option for both weight loss and muscle gain. The lean beef provides protein to support muscle growth, while the cauliflower rice is a low·carb, high·fiber alternative to traditional rice. The vegetables add nutrients and fiber to keep you feeling full and satisfied.

The simple sauce adds flavor without a lot of extra calories or sodium. Enjoy this dish as a complete meal or serve it over a bed of steamed greens for an even more nutrient·dense option.

77. Shrimp and vegetable skewers

Ingredient:

- 1 lb large shrimp, peeled and deveined
- 1 red bell pepper, cut into 1-inch pieces
- 1 yellow bell pepper, cut into 1-inch pieces
- 1 zucchini, cut into 1-inch pieces
- 1 red onion, cut into 1-inch pieces

- 2 tbsp olive oil
- 2 tbsp lemon juice
- 1 tsp dried oregano
- 1 tsp garlic powder
- Salt and pepper to taste

Instructions:

1. In a large bowl, combine the shrimp, bell pepper pieces, zucchini pieces, and onion pieces.

2. In a small bowl, whisk together the olive oil, lemon juice, oregano, and garlic powder. Season with salt and pepper.

3. Pour the marinade over the shrimp and vegetables and toss to coat everything evenly.

4. Thread the marinated shrimp and vegetables onto skewers, alternating the ingredients.

5. Preheat grill or grill pan to medium-high heat.

6. Grill the skewers for 8-10 minutes, turning occasionally, until the shrimp are opaque and the vegetables are tender. Serve the grilled shrimp and vegetable skewers immediately.

These skewers are a great option for a healthy, balanced meal. The shrimp provide lean protein, while the vegetables offer fiber, vitamins, and minerals. The simple marinade adds flavor without a lot of extra calories or fat.

This dish can be a good choice for both weight loss and muscle gain when incorporated into an overall healthy diet and exercise routine. The combination of protein, vegetables, and healthy fats supports various fitness goals.

Serve the skewers with a side of quinoa or brown rice for a complete meal, or enjoy them on their own as a nutritious and satisfying main course.

78. Chicken and quinoa stuffed bell peppers

Ingredient:

- 4 bell peppers, halved and seeded
- 1 lb ground chicken
- 1 cup cooked quinoa
- 1 onion, diced
- 2 cloves garlic, minced
- 1 (14.5 oz) can diced tomatoes
- 1 tsp dried oregano
- 1 tsp chili powder
- Salt and pepper to taste
- 1/2 cup shredded mozzarella cheese (optional)

Instructions:

1. Preheat the oven to 375°F.

2. In a large skillet, cook the ground chicken over medium heat until no longer pink, 5•7 minutes. Drain any excess fat.

3. Add the diced onion and minced garlic to the skillet. Cook for 2•3 minutes until the onion is translucent.

4. Stir in the cooked quinoa, diced tomatoes, oregano, chili powder, salt, and pepper. Cook for an additional 5 minutes.

5. Arrange the bell pepper halves in a baking dish. Spoon the chicken and quinoa mixture into the pepper halves.

6. If using, sprinkle the shredded mozzarella cheese over the top of the stuffed peppers. Bake for 20•25 minutes, or until the peppers are tender and the filling is hot. Serve the stuffed peppers warm.

These stuffed bell peppers are a great option for both weight loss and muscle gain. The ground chicken provides lean protein to support muscle growth, while the quinoa offers complex carbs and fiber to help with weight management. The bell peppers are low in calories and high in nutrients.

The optional mozzarella cheese adds a creamy texture, but the dish can also be enjoyed without it for a lower•calorie option. Pair these stuffed peppers with a side salad or roasted vegetables for a complete, balanced meal.

79. Salmon and sweet potato bowl

Ingredient:

- 4 (6 oz) salmon fillets
- 2 medium sweet potatoes, peeled and cubed
- 2 tbsp olive oil, divided
- 1 cup cooked quinoa
- 1 cup baby spinach
- 1 avocado, diced
- 2 tbsp toasted pumpkin seeds
- 2 tbsp lemon juice
- Salt and pepper to taste

Instructions:

1. Preheat the oven to 400°F.

2. Toss the cubed sweet potatoes with 1 tbsp of olive oil and season with salt and pepper. Spread them out on a baking sheet and roast for 20•25 minutes, or until tender and lightly browned.

3. While the sweet potatoes are roasting, heat the remaining 1 tbsp of olive oil in a skillet over medium•high heat. Season the salmon fillets with salt and pepper and add them to the skillet. Cook for 3•4 minutes per side, or until the salmon is cooked through.

4. In a large bowl, combine the cooked quinoa, roasted sweet potatoes, baby spinach, diced avocado, and toasted pumpkin seeds.

5. Drizzle the lemon juice over the bowl and toss everything together gently.

6. Divide the quinoa and vegetable mixture evenly among 4 bowls. Top each bowl with a salmon fillet. Serve immediately.

This salmon and sweet potato bowl is a nutrient•dense meal that can support both weight loss and muscle gain. The salmon provides lean protein and healthy omega•3 fatty acids, while the sweet potatoes, quinoa, and avocado offer complex carbs, fiber, and healthy fats.

The combination of macronutrients and nutrients in this dish makes it a well•balanced option that can be incorporated into a healthy diet and exercise routine to help achieve your fitness goals.

80. Grilled vegetable and chickpea salad

Ingredient:

- 1 zucchini, sliced
- 1 yellow squash, sliced
- 1 red bell pepper, sliced
- 1 red onion, sliced
- 1 (15 oz) can chickpeas, drained and rinsed
- 2 tbsp olive oil
- 2 tbsp balsamic vinegar
- 1 tsp Dijon mustard
- 1 clove garlic, minced
- 2 tbsp chopped fresh basil
- Salt and pepper to taste

Instructions:

1. Preheat grill or grill pan to medium·high heat.

2. Toss the sliced zucchini, yellow squash, bell pepper, and onion with 1 tbsp of olive oil. Season with salt and pepper.

3. Grill the vegetables for 5·7 minutes per side, or until they are tender and slightly charred.

4. In a large bowl, combine the grilled vegetables and drained, rinsed chickpeas.

5. In a small bowl, whisk together the remaining 1 tbsp of olive oil, balsamic vinegar, Dijon mustard, and minced garlic.

6. Pour the dressing over the grilled vegetables and chickpeas. Toss to coat everything evenly. Sprinkle the chopped fresh basil over the salad and toss again.
Serve the grilled vegetable and chickpea salad warm or at room temperature.

This salad is a great option for both weight loss and muscle gain. The chickpeas provide plant·based protein, while the grilled vegetables offer fiber, vitamins, and minerals. The healthy fats from the olive oil and the complex carbs from the chickpeas and vegetables make this a well·balanced dish.

The simple dressing adds flavor without a lot of extra calories or sodium. Enjoy this salad as a main course or as a side dish to complement a lean protein like grilled chicken or fish.

81. Turkey and vegetable stir·fry

Ingredient:

- 1 lb ground turkey
- 2 tbsp olive oil
- 1 onion, sliced
- 3 cloves garlic, minced
- 1 red bell pepper, sliced
- 1 cup broccoli florets
- 1 cup sliced mushrooms

- 2 cups chopped kale or spinach
- 2 tbsp low·sodium soy sauce
- 1 tbsp rice vinegar
- 1 tsp sesame oil
- Salt and pepper to taste
- Chopped green onions for garnish (optional)

Instructions:

1. In a large skillet or wok, heat the olive oil over medium·high heat.

2. Add the ground turkey and cook, breaking it up with a spatula, until it's no longer pink, about 5·7 minutes. Transfer the turkey to a plate and set aside.

3. Add the sliced onion to the skillet and cook for 2·3 minutes until translucent.

4. Add the minced garlic, sliced bell pepper, broccoli florets, and sliced mushrooms. Stir·fry for 4·5 minutes until the vegetables are tender·crisp.

5. Add the chopped kale or spinach to the skillet and cook for 1·2 minutes until wilted.

6. Return the cooked turkey to the skillet. Stir in the soy sauce, rice vinegar, and sesame oil. Toss everything together until well combined.

7. Season with salt and pepper to taste. Serve the turkey and vegetable stir·fry immediately, garnished with chopped green onions if desired.

This stir·fry is a great option for both weight loss and muscle gain. The ground turkey provides lean protein to support muscle growth, while the vegetables are low in calories and high in fiber, vitamins, and minerals.

The simple sauce adds flavor without a lot of extra calories or sodium. Serve this dish over a bed of steamed brown rice or quinoa for a complete, balanced meal that can support your fitness goals when incorporated into a healthy diet and exercise routine.

82. Beef and vegetable stew

Ingredient:

• 1 lb lean beef stew meat,
cut into 1•inch cubes
• 2 tbsp olive oil
• 1 onion, diced
• 1 tsp dried rosemary
• Salt and pepper to taste
• Chopped parsley for garnish (optional)

• 3 cloves garlic, minced
• 2 carrots, peeled and diced
• 2 celery stalks, diced
• 1 (14.5 oz) can diced tomatoes
• 4 cups low•sodium beef or vegetable broth
• 2 medium potatoes, peeled and cubed
• 1 cup frozen peas
• 1 tsp dried thyme

Instructions:

1. In a large pot or Dutch oven, heat the olive oil over medium•high heat.

2. Add the cubed beef and brown on all sides, about 5•7 minutes. Remove the beef from the pot and set aside.

3. Add the diced onion and minced garlic to the pot. Cook for 2•3 minutes until the onion is translucent.

4. Stir in the diced carrots and celery. Cook for an additional 5 minutes.

5. Pour in the diced tomatoes and beef broth. Add the cubed potatoes, frozen peas, dried thyme, and dried rosemary.

6. Return the browned beef to the pot and bring the stew to a simmer.

7. Reduce heat to medium•low, cover, and let the stew simmer for 45•60 minutes, or until the beef and vegetables are tender.

8. Season with salt and pepper to taste. Serve the beef and vegetable stew hot, garnished with chopped parsley if desired.

This hearty stew is a great option for both weight loss and muscle gain. The lean beef provides protein to support muscle growth, while the vegetables and potatoes offer complex carbs, fiber, and a variety of vitamins and minerals.

The simple seasoning allows the natural flavors of the ingredients to shine through. Enjoy this stew on its own or serve it with a side of crusty whole•grain bread for a complete, balanced meal.

83. Grilled shrimp and vegetable salad

Ingredient:

- 1 red onion, sliced
- 8 cups mixed greens
- 1 avocado, diced
- 2 tbsp balsamic vinegar
- 1 tsp Dijon mustard
- Salt and pepper to taste

- 1 lb large shrimp, peeled and deveined
- 2 tbsp olive oil, divided
- 1 zucchini, sliced
- 1 yellow squash, sliced
- 1 red bell pepper, sliced

Instructions:

1. Preheat grill or grill pan to medium•high heat.

2. In a large bowl, toss the shrimp with 1 tbsp of olive oil and season with salt and pepper.

3. Toss the sliced zucchini, yellow squash, bell pepper, and onion with the remaining 1 tbsp of olive oil and season with salt and pepper.

4. Grill the shrimp for 2•3 minutes per side, or until they are opaque and cooked through. Grill the vegetables for 5•7 minutes per side, or until they are tender and slightly charred.

5. In a large salad bowl, arrange the mixed greens. Top with the grilled shrimp, grilled vegetables, and diced avocado.

6. In a small bowl, whisk together the balsamic vinegar and Dijon mustard. Drizzle the dressing over the salad.

7. Toss the salad gently to coat everything with the dressing. Serve the grilled shrimp and vegetable salad immediately.

This salad is a great option for both weight loss and muscle gain. The grilled shrimp provide lean protein to support muscle growth, while the grilled vegetables and mixed greens are low in calories and high in fiber, vitamins, and minerals.

The healthy fats from the avocado and the simple balsamic vinaigrette dressing add flavor without a lot of extra calories or sodium. This dish can be a satisfying and nutritious main course or a side salad to complement a lean protein.

84. Chicken and vegetable kebabs

Ingredient:

- 1 lb boneless, skinless chicken breasts, cut into 1·inch cubes
- 1 red bell pepper, cut into 1·inch pieces
- 1 yellow bell pepper, cut into 1·inch pieces
- 1 zucchini, cut into 1·inch pieces
- 1 red onion, cut into 1·inch pieces
- 2 tbsp olive oil
- 2 tbsp balsamic vinegar
- 1 tsp dried oregano
- 1 tsp garlic powder
- Salt and pepper to taste

Instructions:

1. In a large bowl, combine the cubed chicken, bell pepper pieces, zucchini pieces, and onion pieces.

2. In a small bowl, whisk together the olive oil, balsamic vinegar, oregano, and garlic powder. Season with salt and pepper.

3. Pour the marinade over the chicken and vegetables and toss to coat everything evenly.

4. Thread the marinated chicken and vegetables onto skewers, alternating the ingredients. Preheat grill or grill pan to medium·high heat.

5. Grill the kebabs for 12·15 minutes, turning occasionally, until the chicken is cooked through and the vegetables are tender. Serve the grilled chicken and vegetable kebabs immediately.

These kebabs are a great option for both weight loss and muscle gain. The chicken provides lean protein to support muscle growth, while the vegetables are low in calories and high in fiber, vitamins, and minerals.

The simple marinade adds flavor without a lot of extra calories or fat. Pair these kebabs with a side of quinoa or brown rice for a complete, balanced meal that can support your fitness goals when incorporated into a healthy diet and exercise routine.

The combination of protein, complex carbs, and nutrient·dense vegetables makes this a versatile and nutritious dish for various fitness objectives.

85. Turkey and quinoa bowl

Ingredient:

- 4 oz cooked turkey breast, diced
- 1/2 cup cooked quinoa
- 1/2 cup diced bell peppers
- 1/4 cup diced onions
- 1 tbsp olive oil
- 1 tsp dried oregano
- Salt and pepper to taste

Instructions:

1. Cook the quinoa according to package instructions. Set aside.

2. In a skillet, heat the olive oil over medium heat. Add the diced onions and bell peppers. Sauté for 5•7 minutes until softened.

3. Add the diced turkey and sauté for another 2•3 minutes until heated through.

4. Stir in the cooked quinoa and oregano. Season with salt and pepper to taste.

5. Serve the turkey and quinoa mixture in a bowl.

Nutritional Information (per serving):

Calories: 280
Protein: 25g
Carbs: 25g
Fat: 10g
Fiber: 4g

This recipe is a great option for weight loss and muscle gain for a few reasons:

1. Turkey is a lean protein source that is low in calories but high in protein, which helps support muscle growth and maintenance.
2. Quinoa is a complex carbohydrate that provides sustained energy and fiber to keep you feeling full.
3. The vegetables add important vitamins, minerals, and antioxidants.
4. The dish is well•balanced with a good ratio of protein, carbs, and healthy fats.

86. Salmon and vegetable stir·fry

Ingredient:

- 1 lb salmon fillets, cut into 1·inch pieces
- 2 tbsp olive oil
- 1 red bell pepper, sliced
- 1 cup broccoli florets
- 1 cup sliced mushrooms
- 2 cups chopped kale or spinach
- 2 tbsp low·sodium soy sauce
- 1 tbsp rice vinegar
- 1 tsp sesame oil
- 2 cloves garlic, minced
- 1 tsp grated ginger
- Salt and pepper to taste
- Chopped green onions for garnish (optional)

Instructions:

1. In a large skillet or wok, heat the olive oil over medium·high heat.

2. Add the salmon pieces and stir·fry for 2·3 minutes until lightly browned. Transfer the salmon to a plate and set aside.

3. Add the sliced bell pepper, broccoli florets, and sliced mushrooms to the skillet. Stir·fry for 4·5 minutes until the vegetables are tender·crisp.

4. Add the chopped kale or spinach to the skillet and cook for 1·2 minutes until wilted.

5. Return the cooked salmon to the skillet. Stir in the soy sauce, rice vinegar, sesame oil, minced garlic, and grated ginger. Toss everything together until well combined.

6. Season with salt and pepper to taste.

7. Serve the salmon and vegetable stir·fry immediately, garnished with chopped green onions if desired.

This stir·fry is a great option for a healthy, balanced meal. The salmon provides lean protein and healthy omega·3 fatty acids, while the vegetables offer fiber, vitamins, and minerals.

The simple sauce adds flavor without a lot of extra calories or sodium. Serve this dish over a bed of steamed brown rice or quinoa for a complete meal that can support both weight loss and muscle gain when incorporated into an overall healthy diet and exercise routine.

87. Grilled chicken and quinoa salad

Ingredient:

- 4 (6 oz) boneless, skinless chicken breasts
- 1 cup cooked quinoa
- 1 cup cherry tomatoes, halved
- 1 cucumber, diced
- 1 avocado, diced
- 1/4 cup crumbled feta cheese
- 2 tbsp olive oil
- 2 tbsp lemon juice
- 1 tsp Dijon mustard
- 1 clove garlic, minced
- Salt and pepper to taste
- Chopped fresh parsley for garnish (optional)

Instructions:

1. Preheat grill or grill pan to medium•high heat.

2. Season the chicken breasts with salt and pepper.

3. Grill the chicken for 5•7 minutes per side, or until it's cooked through and reaches an internal temperature of 165°F. Allow the chicken to rest for 5 minutes, then slice or shred it.

4. In a large bowl, combine the cooked quinoa, halved cherry tomatoes, diced cucumber, diced avocado, and crumbled feta cheese.

5. In a small bowl, whisk together the olive oil, lemon juice, Dijon mustard, and minced garlic. Season with salt and pepper.

6. Pour the dressing over the quinoa salad and toss to coat everything evenly.

7. Add the grilled, sliced or shredded chicken to the salad and gently toss to combine.

8. Serve the grilled chicken and quinoa salad immediately, garnished with chopped fresh parsley if desired.

This salad is a great option for both weight loss and muscle gain. The grilled chicken provides lean protein to support muscle growth, while the quinoa, vegetables, and avocado offer complex carbs, fiber, and healthy fats.

The simple dressing adds flavor without a lot of extra calories or sodium. This dish can be a satisfying and nutritious main course or a side salad to complement a lean protein•based meal.

88. Beef and broccoli bowl

Ingredient:

- 1 lb flank steak, thinly sliced
- 3 cups broccoli florets
- 2 tbsp low•sodium soy sauce
- 1 tbsp rice vinegar
- 1 tsp sesame oil
- 1 tsp cornstarch
- 2 tbsp olive oil
- 3 cloves garlic, minced
- 1 tbsp grated ginger
- 2 cups cooked brown rice
- Chopped green onions for garnish (optional)

Instructions:

1. In a small bowl, whisk together the soy sauce, rice vinegar, sesame oil, and cornstarch. Set aside.

2. Heat the olive oil in a large skillet or wok over high heat.

3. Add the thinly sliced flank steak and stir•fry for 2•3 minutes until lightly browned.

4. Add the minced garlic and grated ginger to the skillet. Cook for 1 minute, stirring constantly.

5. Add the broccoli florets to the skillet and stir•fry for 3•4 minutes until the broccoli is tender•crisp.

6. Pour the soy sauce mixture into the skillet and toss everything together. Cook for 2•3 minutes, or until the sauce has thickened.

7. Remove from heat and serve the beef and broccoli over the cooked brown rice. Garnish with chopped green onions if desired.

This beef and broccoli bowl is a great option for both weight loss and muscle gain. The flank steak provides lean protein to support muscle growth, while the broccoli is low in calories and high in fiber, vitamins, and minerals.

The simple sauce adds flavor without a lot of extra calories or sodium. Serving the dish over brown rice provides complex carbs to fuel your workouts and support overall health.

This balanced meal can be a great addition to a healthy diet and exercise routine aimed at achieving your fitness goals, whether that's weight loss, muscle gain, or overall wellness.

89. Shrimp and vegetable curry

Ingredient:

- 1 lb peeled and deveined shrimp
- 1 tbsp olive oil
- 1 onion, diced
- 3 cloves garlic, minced
- 1 tbsp grated ginger
- 2 tsp curry powder
- 1 tsp ground cumin
- 1 tsp ground coriander
- 1 tsp turmeric
- 1 cup diced tomatoes
- 1 cup low•sodium vegetable or chicken broth
- 1 cup diced cauliflower
- 1 cup diced zucchini
- 1/2 cup full•fat coconut milk
- Salt and pepper to taste
- Chopped cilantro for garnish

Instructions:

1. In a large skillet or wok, heat the olive oil over medium heat. Add the onion and sauté for 3•4 minutes until translucent.

2. Add the garlic and ginger and sauté for 1 minute until fragrant.

3. Stir in the curry powder, cumin, coriander, and turmeric. Cook for 1 minute to toast the spices.

4. Pour in the diced tomatoes and broth. Bring to a simmer.

5. Add the cauliflower and zucchini. Simmer for 5•7 minutes until the vegetables are tender.

6. Stir in the shrimp and coconut milk. Cook for 3•5 minutes until the shrimp are opaque and cooked through.

7. Season with salt and pepper to taste. Serve the curry over steamed rice or quinoa. Garnish with chopped cilantro.

This curry is a great option for a healthy, balanced meal. The shrimp provides lean protein, while the vegetables and coconut milk add fiber, vitamins, and healthy fats. Adjust the spices to your desired level of heat. Enjoy!

90. Chicken and vegetable skewers

Ingredient:

- 1 lb boneless, skinless chicken breasts, cut into 1•inch cubes
- 1 red bell pepper, cut into 1•inch pieces
- 1 zucchini, cut into 1•inch pieces
- 1 red onion, cut into 1•inch pieces
- 8 oz mushrooms, halved
- 2 tbsp olive oil
- 2 tsp dried oregano
- 1 tsp garlic powder
- Salt and pepper to taste

Instructions:

1. Preheat grill or grill pan to medium•high heat.

2. In a large bowl, toss the chicken, bell pepper, zucchini, onion, and mushrooms with the olive oil, oregano, garlic powder, salt, and pepper until evenly coated.

3. Thread the chicken and vegetables onto skewers, alternating the ingredients. Grill the skewers for 12•15 minutes, turning occasionally, until the chicken is cooked through and the vegetables are tender.

Nutritional Information (per serving, 2 skewers):
Calories: 250
Protein: 30g
Carbs: 12g
Fat: 10g
Fiber: 3g

This recipe is great for weight loss and muscle gain for a few reasons:
1. Chicken is a lean protein source that helps build and maintain muscle mass.
2. The vegetables provide fiber, vitamins, minerals, and antioxidants to support overall health.
3. The dish is relatively low in calories but high in protein and nutrients, making it a filling and satisfying meal.
4. Grilling the skewers adds a nice smoky flavor without needing to use high•calorie sauces or dressings.

You can adjust the portion sizes as needed to fit your specific calorie and macronutrient goals. Serve the skewers over a bed of greens or with a side of roasted sweet potatoes for a complete, balanced meal. Enjoy!

91. Turkey and sweet potato bowl

Ingredient:

- 1 lb ground turkey
- 1 medium sweet potato, diced
- 1 cup diced bell peppers
- 1/2 cup diced onion
- 2 cloves garlic, minced
- 1 tsp chili powder
- 1 tsp cumin
- 1/2 tsp paprika
- Salt and pepper to taste
- 2 cups baby spinach
- 1/4 cup crumbled feta cheese

Instructions:

1. Preheat oven to 400°F. Toss the diced sweet potato with 1 tbsp olive oil and season with salt and pepper. Spread on a baking sheet and roast for 20•25 minutes, until tender.

2. In a large skillet over medium•high heat, cook the ground turkey, breaking it up with a spatula, until browned and cooked through, about 5•7 minutes. Drain any excess fat.

3. Add the diced bell peppers, onion, and garlic to the skillet with the turkey. Sauté for 3•4 minutes until the vegetables are softened.

4. Stir in the chili powder, cumin, paprika, and season with salt and pepper to taste.

5. To assemble the bowls, divide the roasted sweet potato, turkey•vegetable mixture, and baby spinach evenly among 4 bowls. Top each bowl with 1 tbsp of crumbled feta cheese.

This turkey and sweet potato bowl is an excellent choice for weight loss and muscle gain for several reasons:

1. Ground turkey is a lean protein source that helps build and maintain muscle mass.
2. Sweet potatoes are a complex carbohydrate that provides sustained energy and fiber to keep you feeling full.
3. The vegetables add important vitamins, minerals, and antioxidants to support overall health.

92. Grilled salmon and vegetable salad

Ingredient:

- 4 (4 oz) salmon fillets
- 2 tbsp olive oil, divided
- 1 tsp lemon pepper seasoning
- 4 cups mixed greens
- 1 cup cherry tomatoes, halved
- 1 cucumber, sliced
- 1/2 red onion, thinly sliced
- 1/4 cup crumbled feta cheese
- 2 tbsp balsamic vinegar
- Salt and pepper to taste

Instructions:

1. Preheat grill or grill pan to medium•high heat.

2. Brush the salmon fillets with 1 tbsp of the olive oil and season with the lemon pepper seasoning.

3. Grill the salmon for 4•6 minutes per side, until cooked through. Set aside.

4. In a large salad bowl, combine the mixed greens, cherry tomatoes, cucumber, and red onion.

5. Drizzle the remaining 1 tbsp olive oil and the balsamic vinegar over the salad. Toss to coat.

6. Top the salad with the grilled salmon fillets and crumbled feta cheese.Season with salt and pepper to taste.

This salad is an excellent choice for weight loss and muscle gain for several reasons:

1. Salmon is a high•quality, lean protein that helps build and maintain muscle mass.
2. The vegetables provide fiber, vitamins, minerals, and antioxidants to support overall health and weight management.
3. The healthy fats from the salmon and olive oil help keep you feeling full and satisfied.
4. The dish is relatively low in calories but high in nutrients, making it a filling and nutritious meal.

93. Chicken and quinoa stir·fry

Ingredient:

- 1 lb boneless, skinless chicken breasts, cut into 1·inch pieces
- 1 cup cooked quinoa
- 2 cups mixed vegetables (such as broccoli, bell peppers, snap peas, carrots)
- 2 tbsp low·sodium soy sauce
- 1 tbsp rice vinegar
- 1 tsp sesame oil
- 2 cloves garlic, minced
- 1 tsp grated ginger
- 1 tbsp olive oil
- Salt and pepper to taste
- Chopped green onions for garnish (optional)

Instructions:

1. In a large skillet or wok, heat the olive oil over medium·high heat.

2. Add the chicken and stir·fry for 5·7 minutes until cooked through and no longer pink.

3. Add the mixed vegetables and stir·fry for another 3·4 minutes until the vegetables are tender·crisp.

4. Stir in the cooked quinoa, soy sauce, rice vinegar, sesame oil, garlic, and ginger. Toss everything together and cook for 2·3 minutes until heated through.

5. Season with salt and pepper to taste.

6. Serve the chicken and quinoa stir·fry hot, garnished with chopped green onions if desired.

This chicken and quinoa stir·fry is an excellent choice for weight loss and muscle gain for several reasons:

1. Chicken is a lean protein source that helps build and maintain muscle mass.
2. Quinoa is a high·protein, high·fiber complex carbohydrate that provides sustained energy.
3. The vegetables add important vitamins, minerals, and antioxidants to support overall health.
4. The dish is relatively low in calories but high in nutrients, making it a filling and satisfying meal.

94. Beef and vegetable chili

Ingredient:

- 1 lb lean ground beef
- 1 onion, diced
- 3 cloves garlic, minced
- 1 bell pepper, diced
- 1 zucchini, diced
- 1 can (15 oz) diced tomatoes
- 1 can (15 oz) kidney beans, rinsed and drained
- 2 tbsp chili powder
- 1 tsp cumin
- 1 tsp oregano
- 1/2 tsp smoked paprika
- Salt and pepper to taste
- Chopped cilantro for garnish (optional)

Instructions:

1. In a large pot or Dutch oven, cook the ground beef over medium·high heat, breaking it up with a wooden spoon, until browned and cooked through, about 5·7 minutes. Drain any excess fat.

2. Add the diced onion and garlic to the pot. Sauté for 2·3 minutes until the onion is translucent.

3. Stir in the diced bell pepper and zucchini. Cook for 5 minutes, stirring occasionally, until the vegetables are slightly softened.

4. Add the diced tomatoes, kidney beans, chili powder, cumin, oregano, and smoked paprika. Stir to combine.

5. Bring the chili to a simmer and let it cook for 15·20 minutes, stirring occasionally, until the flavors have melded and the vegetables are tender.

6. Season with salt and pepper to taste. Serve the beef and vegetable chili hot, garnished with chopped cilantro if desired.

You can adjust the portion sizes as needed to fit your specific calorie and macronutrient goals. Enjoy this delicious and healthy beef and vegetable chili!

95. Shrimp and vegetable soup

Ingredient:

- 1 lb peeled and deveined shrimp
- 4 cups low•sodium chicken or vegetable broth
- 1 cup diced onion
- 1 cup diced carrots
- 1 cup diced celery
- 1 cup diced zucchini
- 2 cloves garlic, minced
- 1 tsp dried thyme
- 1 tsp dried oregano
- Salt and pepper to taste
- Chopped parsley for garnish (optional)

Instructions:

1. In a large pot or Dutch oven, bring the broth to a simmer over medium heat.

2. Add the diced onion, carrots, celery, and zucchini to the pot. Simmer for 10•12 minutes, until the vegetables are tender.

3. Stir in the minced garlic, dried thyme, and dried oregano. Cook for 1•2 minutes until fragrant.

4. Add the shrimp to the pot and continue simmering for 5•7 minutes, until the shrimp are opaque and cooked through.

5. Season the soup with salt and pepper to taste. Serve the shrimp and vegetable soup hot, garnished with chopped parsley if desired.

This shrimp and vegetable soup is an excellent choice for weight loss and muscle gain for several reasons:

1. Shrimp is a lean protein source that helps build and maintain muscle mass.
2. The vegetables add fiber, vitamins, minerals, and antioxidants to support overall health and weight management.
3. The dish is relatively low in calories but high in nutrients, making it a filling and satisfying meal.
4. The broth•based soup provides hydration and a light, comforting texture.

96. Chicken and vegetable stew

Ingredient:

- 1 lb boneless, skinless chicken breasts, cut into 1•inch pieces
- 2 tbsp olive oil
- 1 onion, diced
- 3 cloves garlic, minced
- 2 carrots, peeled and diced
- 2 celery stalks, diced
- 1 cup diced potatoes
- 1 cup diced zucchini
- 4 cups low•sodium chicken broth
- 1 tsp dried thyme
- 1 tsp dried rosemary
- Salt and pepper to taste
- Chopped parsley for garnish (optional)

Instructions:

1. In a large pot or Dutch oven, heat the olive oil over medium•high heat. Add the chicken and cook for 3•4 minutes, until lightly browned on the outside.

2. Add the diced onion and garlic to the pot. Sauté for 2•3 minutes until the onion is translucent.

3. Stir in the diced carrots, celery, potatoes, and zucchini. Cook for 5 minutes, stirring occasionally.

4. Pour in the chicken broth and add the dried thyme and rosemary. Season with salt and pepper to taste.

5. Bring the stew to a boil, then reduce the heat and let it simmer for 20•25 minutes, until the vegetables are tender and the chicken is cooked through.

6. Serve the chicken and vegetable stew hot, garnished with chopped parsley if desired.

You can adjust the portion sizes as needed to fit your specific calorie and macronutrient goals. Enjoy this delicious and healthy chicken and vegetable stew!

97. Grilled turkey and vegetable kebabs

Ingredient:

- 1 lb ground turkey, formed into 1-inch meatballs
- 1 red bell pepper, cut into 1-inch pieces
- 1 zucchini, cut into 1-inch pieces
- 1 red onion, cut into 1-inch pieces
- 8 oz mushrooms, halved
- 2 tbsp olive oil
- 1 tsp dried oregano
- 1 tsp garlic powder
- Salt and pepper to taste
- Wooden or metal skewers

Instructions:

1. Preheat grill or grill pan to medium-high heat.

2. In a large bowl, toss the turkey meatballs, bell pepper, zucchini, onion, and mushrooms with the olive oil, oregano, garlic powder, salt, and pepper until evenly coated.

3. Thread the turkey meatballs and vegetables onto the skewers, alternating the ingredients.

4. Grill the kebabs for 12-15 minutes, turning occasionally, until the turkey is cooked through and the vegetables are tender.

This recipe for grilled turkey and vegetable kebabs is an excellent choice for weight loss and muscle gain for several reasons:

1. Ground turkey is a lean protein source that helps build and maintain muscle mass.
2. The vegetables provide fiber, vitamins, minerals, and antioxidants to support overall health and weight management.
3. The dish is relatively low in calories but high in protein and nutrients, making it a filling and satisfying meal.
4. Grilling the kebabs adds a nice smoky flavor without needing to use high-calorie sauces or dressings.

You can adjust the portion sizes as needed to fit your specific calorie and macronutrient goals. Serve the kebabs over a bed of greens or with a side of roasted sweet potatoes for a complete, balanced meal. Enjoy!

98. Salmon and broccoli stir·fry

Ingredient:

- 1 lb salmon fillets, cut into 1·inch pieces
- 2 cups broccoli florets
- 1 red bell pepper, sliced
- 1 cup sliced mushrooms
- 2 cloves garlic, minced
- 1 tbsp grated ginger
- 2 tbsp low·sodium soy sauce
- 1 tbsp rice vinegar
- 1 tsp sesame oil
- 1 tbsp olive oil
- Salt and pepper to taste
- Chopped green onions for garnish (optional)

Instructions:

1. In a large skillet or wok, heat the olive oil over medium·high heat.

2. Add the salmon pieces and stir·fry for 2·3 minutes until lightly browned on the outside.

3. Add the broccoli florets, bell pepper slices, and mushrooms to the skillet. Stir·fry for 3·4 minutes until the vegetables are tender·crisp.

4. Stir in the minced garlic and grated ginger. Cook for 1 minute until fragrant.

5. Pour in the soy sauce, rice vinegar, and sesame oil. Toss everything together and cook for 2·3 minutes until the sauce has thickened slightly.

6. Season with salt and pepper to taste. Serve the salmon and broccoli stir·fry hot, garnished with chopped green onions if desired.

Nutritional Information (per serving):
Calories: 300
Protein: 30g
Carbs: 12g
Fat: 15g
Fiber: 4g

You can adjust the portion sizes as needed to fit your specific calorie and macronutrient goals. Enjoy this delicious and healthy salmon and broccoli stir·fry!

99. Chicken and sweet potato curry

Ingredient:

- 1 lb boneless, skinless chicken breasts, cut into 1-inch pieces
- 2 medium sweet potatoes, peeled and diced
- 1 onion, diced
- 3 cloves garlic, minced
- 1 tbsp grated ginger
- 2 tsp curry powder
- 1 tsp ground cumin
- 1 tsp ground coriander
- 1 tsp turmeric
- 1 cup low-sodium chicken broth
- 1 cup full-fat coconut milk
- Salt and pepper to taste
- Chopped cilantro for garnish (optional)

Instructions:

1. In a large skillet or Dutch oven, heat 1 tbsp of olive oil over medium-high heat.

2. Add the diced chicken and sauté for 3-4 minutes until lightly browned.

3. Add the diced onion and sauté for 2-3 minutes until translucent.

4. Stir in the minced garlic and grated ginger. Cook for 1 minute until fragrant.

5. Add the curry powder, cumin, coriander, and turmeric. Stir to coat the chicken and vegetables.

6. Pour in the chicken broth and coconut milk. Bring the mixture to a simmer.

7. Add the diced sweet potatoes and season with salt and pepper to taste.

8. Reduce the heat to medium-low and let the curry simmer for 15-20 minutes, until the sweet potatoes are tender and the sauce has thickened.

9. Serve the chicken and sweet potato curry hot, garnished with chopped cilantro if desired.

You can adjust the portion sizes as needed to fit your specific calorie and macronutrient goals. Enjoy this delicious and healthy chicken and sweet potato curry!

100. Turkey and quinoa stir·fry

Ingredient:

- 1 lb ground turkey
- 1 cup cooked quinoa
- 2 cups mixed vegetables (such as broccoli, bell peppers, snap peas, carrots)
- 2 tbsp low·sodium soy sauce
- 1 tbsp rice vinegar
- 1 tsp sesame oil
- 2 cloves garlic, minced
- 1 tsp grated ginger
- 1 tbsp olive oil
- Salt and pepper to taste
- Chopped green onions for garnish (optional)

Instructions:

1. In a large skillet or wok, heat the olive oil over medium·high heat.

2. Add the ground turkey and stir·fry for 5·7 minutes until cooked through and no longer pink.

3. Add the mixed vegetables and stir·fry for another 3·4 minutes until the vegetables are tender·crisp.

4. Stir in the cooked quinoa, soy sauce, rice vinegar, sesame oil, garlic, and ginger. Toss everything together and cook for 2·3 minutes until heated through.

5. Season with salt and pepper to taste. Serve the turkey and quinoa stir·fry hot, garnished with chopped green onions if desired.

Nutritional Information (per serving):
Calories: 350
Protein: 35g
Carbs: 30g
Fat: 12g
Fiber: 5g

You can adjust the portion sizes as needed to fit your specific calorie and macronutrient goals. Enjoy this delicious and healthy turkey and quinoa stir·fry!

101. Beef and vegetable skillet

Ingredient:

- 1 lb lean ground beef
- 1 onion, diced
- 3 cloves garlic, minced
- 1 cup diced bell peppers
- 1 cup diced zucchini
- 1 cup diced mushrooms
- 1 can (15 oz) diced tomatoes
- 2 tsp dried oregano
- 1 tsp dried basil
- Salt and pepper to taste
- Chopped parsley for garnish (optional)

Instructions:

1. In a large skillet or cast·iron pan, cook the ground beef over medium·high heat, breaking it up with a wooden spoon, until browned and cooked through, about 5·7 minutes. Drain any excess fat.

2. Add the diced onion and garlic to the skillet. Sauté for 2·3 minutes until the onion is translucent.

3. Stir in the diced bell peppers, zucchini, and mushrooms. Cook for 5·7 minutes, stirring occasionally, until the vegetables are tender.

4. Pour in the diced tomatoes and add the dried oregano and basil. Stir to combine.

5. Season the beef and vegetable mixture with salt and pepper to taste.

6. Reduce the heat to medium·low and let the skillet simmer for 10·15 minutes, allowing the flavors to meld.

7. Serve the beef and vegetable skillet hot, garnished with chopped parsley if desired.

You can adjust the portion sizes as needed to fit your specific calorie and macronutrient goals. Enjoy this delicious and healthy beef and vegetable skillet!

102. Shrimp and vegetable stir·fry

Ingredient:

- 1 lb peeled and deveined shrimp
- 2 tbsp olive oil
- 2 cups mixed vegetables (such as broccoli, bell peppers, snap peas, carrots)
- 2 cloves garlic, minced
- 1 tbsp grated ginger
- 2 tbsp low·sodium soy sauce
- 1 tbsp rice vinegar
- 1 tsp sesame oil
- Salt and pepper to taste
- Chopped green onions for garnish (optional)

Instructions:

1. In a large skillet or wok, heat the olive oil over medium·high heat.

2. Add the shrimp and stir·fry for 2·3 minutes until they start to turn pink.

3. Add the mixed vegetables and continue stir·frying for 3·4 minutes until the vegetables are tender·crisp.

4. Stir in the minced garlic and grated ginger. Cook for 1 minute until fragrant.

5. Pour in the soy sauce, rice vinegar, and sesame oil. Toss everything together and cook for 2·3 minutes until the sauce has thickened slightly.

6. Season with salt and pepper to taste.

7. Serve the shrimp and vegetable stir·fry hot, garnished with chopped green onions if desired.

You can adjust the portion sizes as needed to fit your specific calorie and macronutrient goals. Enjoy this delicious and healthy shrimp and vegetable stir·fry!

103. Chicken and quinoa bowl

Ingredient:

- 1 lb boneless, skinless chicken breasts, grilled or baked and diced
- 1 cup cooked quinoa
- 1 cup diced bell peppers
- 1 cup diced cucumber
- 1/2 cup diced red onion
- 2 tbsp chopped fresh cilantro
- 2 tbsp olive oil
- 1 tbsp lime juice
- 1 tsp ground cumin
- Salt and pepper to taste

Instructions:

1. Cook the quinoa according to package instructions. Set aside to cool.

2. In a large bowl, combine the diced chicken, cooked quinoa, diced bell peppers, cucumber, and red onion.

3. In a small bowl, whisk together the olive oil, lime juice, and ground cumin. Season with salt and pepper to taste.

4. Pour the dressing over the chicken and quinoa mixture and toss to coat evenly.

5. Sprinkle the chopped fresh cilantro over the top.

6. Serve the chicken and quinoa bowl warm or chilled.

Nutritional Information (per serving):
Calories: 350
Protein: 35g
Carbs: 30g
Fat: 12g
Fiber: 5g

You can adjust the portion sizes as needed to fit your specific calorie and macronutrient goals. Enjoy this delicious and healthy chicken and quinoa bowl!

104. Grilled salmon and quinoa salad

Ingredient:

- 4 (4 oz) salmon fillets
- 1 cup cooked quinoa
- 2 cups mixed greens
- 1 cup cherry tomatoes, halved
- 1/2 cup diced cucumber
- 1/4 cup crumbled feta cheese
- 2 tbsp olive oil
- 1 tbsp balsamic vinegar
- 1 tsp Dijon mustard
- 1 tsp honey
- Salt and pepper to taste

Instructions:

1. Preheat grill or grill pan to medium•high heat.

2. Season the salmon fillets with salt and pepper.

3. Grill the salmon for 4•6 minutes per side, until cooked through. Set aside.

4. In a large salad bowl, combine the cooked quinoa, mixed greens, cherry tomatoes, and diced cucumber.

5. In a small bowl, whisk together the olive oil, balsamic vinegar, Dijon mustard, and honey. Season with salt and pepper.

6. Drizzle the dressing over the quinoa salad and toss to coat.

7. Top the salad with the grilled salmon fillets and crumbled feta cheese.

Nutritional Information (per serving):
Calories: 350
Protein: 30g
Carbs: 25g
Fat: 15g
Fiber: 5g

You can adjust the portion sizes as needed to fit your specific calorie and macronutrient goals. Enjoy this delicious and healthy grilled salmon and quinoa salad!

105. Turkey and vegetable soup

Ingredient:

- 1 lb ground turkey
- 1 onion, diced
- 3 cloves garlic, minced
- 4 cups low•sodium chicken or vegetable broth
- 2 cups diced carrots
- 2 cups diced celery
- 1 cup diced zucchini
- 1 cup diced green beans
- 1 tsp dried thyme
- 1 tsp dried oregano
- Salt and pepper to taste
- Chopped parsley for garnish (optional)

Instructions:

1. In a large pot or Dutch oven, cook the ground turkey over medium•high heat, breaking it up with a wooden spoon, until browned and cooked through, about 5•7 minutes. Drain any excess fat.

2. Add the diced onion and garlic to the pot. Sauté for 2•3 minutes until the onion is translucent.

3. Pour in the chicken or vegetable broth and add the diced carrots, celery, zucchini, and green beans.

4. Stir in the dried thyme and oregano. Season with salt and pepper to taste.

5. Bring the soup to a boil, then reduce the heat and let it simmer for 20•25 minutes, until the vegetables are tender. Serve the turkey and vegetable soup hot, garnished with chopped parsley if desired.

Nutritional Information (per serving):
Calories: 250
Protein: 25g
Carbs: 15g
Fat: 8g
Fiber: 4g

You can adjust the portion sizes as needed to fit your specific calorie and macronutrient goals. Enjoy this delicious and healthy turkey and vegetable soup!

106. Chicken and vegetable kebabs

Ingredient:

- 1 lb boneless, skinless chicken breasts, cut into 1·inch cubes
- 1 red bell pepper, cut into 1·inch pieces
- 1 zucchini, cut into 1·inch pieces
- 1 red onion, cut into 1·inch pieces
- 8 oz mushrooms, halved
- 2 tbsp olive oil
- 1 tsp dried oregano
- 1 tsp garlic powder
- Salt and pepper to taste
- Wooden or metal skewers

Instructions:

1. Preheat grill or grill pan to medium·high heat.

2. In a large bowl, toss the chicken cubes, bell pepper, zucchini, onion, and mushrooms with the olive oil, oregano, garlic powder, salt, and pepper until evenly coated.

3. Thread the chicken and vegetables onto the skewers, alternating the ingredients.

4. Grill the kebabs for 12·15 minutes, turning occasionally, until the chicken is cooked through and the vegetables are tender.

These chicken and vegetable kebabs are an excellent choice for weight loss and muscle gain for several reasons:

1. Chicken is a lean protein source that helps build and maintain muscle mass.
2. The vegetables provide fiber, vitamins, minerals, and antioxidants to support overall health and weight management.
3. The dish is relatively low in calories but high in protein and nutrients, making it a filling and satisfying meal.
4. Grilling the kebabs adds a nice smoky flavor without needing to use high·calorie sauces or dressings.

You can adjust the portion sizes as needed to fit your specific calorie and macronutrient goals. Serve the kebabs over a bed of greens or with a side of roasted sweet potatoes for a complete, balanced meal. Enjoy!

107. Beef and vegetable stir•fry

Ingredient:

- 1 lb lean beef (such as sirloin or flank steak), thinly sliced
- 2 tbsp olive oil
- 2 cups mixed vegetables (such as broccoli, bell peppers, snap peas, carrots)
- 2 cloves garlic, minced
- 1 tbsp grated ginger
- 2 tbsp low•sodium soy sauce
- 1 tbsp rice vinegar
- 1 tsp sesame oil
- Salt and pepper to taste
- Chopped green onions for garnish (optional)

Instructions:

1. In a large skillet or wok, heat the olive oil over medium•high heat.

2. Add the sliced beef and stir•fry for 3•4 minutes until lightly browned.

3. Add the mixed vegetables and stir•fry for another 3•4 minutes until the vegetables are tender•crisp.

4. Stir in the minced garlic and grated ginger. Cook for 1 minute until fragrant.

5. Pour in the soy sauce, rice vinegar, and sesame oil. Toss everything together and cook for 2•3 minutes until the sauce has thickened slightly.

6. Season with salt and pepper to taste.

7. Serve the beef and vegetable stir•fry hot, garnished with chopped green onions if desired.

This beef and vegetable stir•fry is a great option for a healthy, balanced meal. The lean beef provides protein to support muscle growth and maintenance, while the vegetables add fiber, vitamins, and minerals. The combination of protein, complex carbohydrates, and healthy fats helps keep you feeling full and satisfied.

You can adjust the portion sizes as needed to fit your specific calorie and macronutrient goals. Feel free to customize the vegetables based on your preferences. Enjoy this delicious and nutritious beef and vegetable stir•fry!

108. Shrimp and quinoa bowl

Ingredient:

- 1 lb peeled and deveined shrimp
- 1 cup cooked quinoa
- 1 cup diced bell peppers
- 1 cup diced cucumber
- 1/2 cup diced red onion
- 2 tbsp chopped fresh cilantro
- 2 tbsp olive oil
- 1 tbsp lime juice
- 1 tsp ground cumin
- Salt and pepper to taste

Instructions:

1. Cook the quinoa according to package instructions. Set aside to cool.

2. In a large bowl, combine the cooked shrimp, quinoa, diced bell peppers, cucumber, and red onion.

3. In a small bowl, whisk together the olive oil, lime juice, and ground cumin. Season with salt and pepper to taste.

4. Pour the dressing over the shrimp and quinoa mixture and toss to coat evenly.

5. Sprinkle the chopped fresh cilantro over the top.

6. Serve the shrimp and quinoa bowl warm or chilled.

This shrimp and quinoa bowl is a great option for a healthy, balanced meal. The shrimp provides lean protein, while the quinoa is a high•protein, high•fiber complex carbohydrate that provides sustained energy. The vegetables add important vitamins, minerals, and antioxidants.

The combination of protein, complex carbohydrates, and healthy fats helps keep you feeling full and satisfied. You can adjust the portion sizes as needed to fit your specific calorie and macronutrient goals.

Feel free to customize the vegetables based on your preferences. This shrimp and quinoa bowl is a delicious and nutritious meal that can be enjoyed for weight loss or muscle gain.

109. Chicken and sweet potato bowl

Ingredient:

- 1 lb boneless, skinless chicken breasts, grilled or baked and diced
- 2 medium sweet potatoes, diced and roasted
- 1 cup cooked quinoa
- 1 cup diced bell peppers
- 1/2 cup diced red onion
- 2 tbsp chopped fresh parsley
- 2 tbsp olive oil
- 1 tbsp apple cider vinegar
- 1 tsp Dijon mustard
- Salt and pepper to taste

Instructions:

1. Preheat oven to 400°F. Toss the diced sweet potatoes with 1 tbsp olive oil and season with salt and pepper. Spread on a baking sheet and roast for 20•25 minutes, until tender.

2. Cook the quinoa according to package instructions. Set aside to cool.

3. In a large bowl, combine the diced chicken, roasted sweet potatoes, cooked quinoa, diced bell peppers, and diced red onion.

4. In a small bowl, whisk together the remaining 1 tbsp olive oil, apple cider vinegar, and Dijon mustard. Season with salt and pepper to taste.

5. Pour the dressing over the chicken and vegetable mixture and toss to coat evenly. Sprinkle the chopped fresh parsley over the top. Serve the chicken and sweet potato bowl warm or chilled.

The combination of protein, complex carbohydrates, and healthy fats helps keep you feeling full and satisfied. You can adjust the portion sizes as needed to fit your specific calorie and macronutrient goals.

Feel free to customize the vegetables based on your preferences. This chicken and sweet potato bowl is a delicious and nutritious meal that can be enjoyed for weight loss or muscle gain.

110. Turkey and vegetable stew

Ingredient:

- 1 lb ground turkey
- 2 tbsp olive oil
- 1 onion, diced
- 3 cloves garlic, minced
- 2 carrots, peeled and diced
- 2 celery stalks, diced
- 1 cup diced potatoes
- 1 cup diced zucchini
- 4 cups low•sodium chicken broth
- 1 tsp dried thyme
- 1 tsp dried rosemary
- Salt and pepper to taste
- Chopped parsley for garnish (optional)

Instructions:

1. In a large pot or Dutch oven, heat the olive oil over medium•high heat. Add the ground turkey and cook for 5•7 minutes, breaking it up with a wooden spoon, until browned and cooked through.

2. Add the diced onion and garlic to the pot. Sauté for 2•3 minutes until the onion is translucent.

3. Stir in the diced carrots, celery, potatoes, and zucchini. Cook for 5 minutes, stirring occasionally.

4. Pour in the chicken broth and add the dried thyme and rosemary. Season with salt and pepper to taste.

5. Bring the stew to a boil, then reduce the heat and let it simmer for 20•25 minutes, until the vegetables are tender and the flavors have melded. Serve the turkey and vegetable stew hot, garnished with chopped parsley if desired.

This turkey and vegetable stew is a great option for a healthy, comforting meal. The ground turkey provides lean protein, while the vegetables add fiber, vitamins, and minerals. The combination of protein, complex carbohydrates, and healthy fats helps keep you feeling full and satisfied.

You can adjust the portion sizes as needed to fit your specific calorie and macronutrient goals. Feel free to customize the vegetables based on your preferences. This turkey and vegetable stew is a delicious and nutritious meal that can be enjoyed for weight loss or muscle gain.

III. Salmon and vegetable skewers

Ingredient:

- 1 lb salmon fillets, cut into 1-inch cubes
- 1 red bell pepper, cut into 1-inch pieces
- 1 zucchini, cut into 1-inch pieces
- 1 red onion, cut into 1-inch pieces
- 8 oz mushrooms, halved
- 2 tbsp olive oil
- 1 tsp dried dill
- 1 tsp garlic powder
- Salt and pepper to taste
- Wooden or metal skewers

Instructions:

1. Preheat grill or grill pan to medium-high heat.

2. In a large bowl, toss the salmon cubes, bell pepper, zucchini, onion, and mushrooms with the olive oil, dried dill, garlic powder, salt, and pepper until evenly coated.

3. Thread the salmon and vegetables onto the skewers, alternating the ingredients.

4. Grill the skewers for 10-12 minutes, turning occasionally, until the salmon is cooked through and the vegetables are tender.

These salmon and vegetable skewers are a great option for a healthy, balanced meal. The salmon provides lean protein and healthy omega-3 fatty acids, while the vegetables add fiber, vitamins, and minerals.

The combination of protein, complex carbohydrates, and healthy fats helps keep you feeling full and satisfied. You can adjust the portion sizes as needed to fit your specific calorie and macronutrient goals.

Feel free to customize the vegetables based on your preferences. This salmon and vegetable skewer dish is a delicious and nutritious meal that can be enjoyed for weight loss or muscle gain.

112. Grilled chicken and vegetable salad

Ingredient:

- 1 lb boneless, skinless chicken breasts
- 2 cups mixed greens
- 1 cup diced bell peppers
- 1 cup diced cucumber
- 1/2 cup diced red onion
- 1/4 cup crumbled feta cheese
- 2 tbsp olive oil
- 1 tbsp balsamic vinegar
- 1 tsp Dijon mustard
- 1 tsp honey
- Salt and pepper to taste

Instructions:

1. Preheat grill or grill pan to medium•high heat.

2. Season the chicken breasts with salt and pepper.

3. Grill the chicken for 5•7 minutes per side, until cooked through. Let rest for 5 minutes, then slice or dice the chicken.

4. In a large salad bowl, combine the mixed greens, diced bell peppers, cucumber, and red onion.

5. In a small bowl, whisk together the olive oil, balsamic vinegar, Dijon mustard, and honey. Season with salt and pepper to taste.

6. Drizzle the dressing over the salad and toss to coat. Top the salad with the grilled chicken and crumbled feta cheese.

This grilled chicken and vegetable salad is an excellent choice for weight loss and muscle gain for several reasons:

1. Grilled chicken is a lean protein source that helps build and maintain muscle mass.
2. The mixed greens and other vegetables add fiber, vitamins, minerals, and antioxidants to support overall health and weight management.
3. The healthy fats from the olive oil and feta cheese help keep you feeling satisfied.
4. The dish is relatively low in calories but high in nutrients, making it a filling and nutritious meal.

113. Beef and quinoa bowl

Ingredient:

- 1 lb ground beef
- 1 cup uncooked quinoa, rinsed
- 2 cups low•sodium beef broth
- 1 cup diced tomatoes
- 1 cup diced bell pepper
- 1/2 cup diced onion
- 2 cloves garlic, minced
- 1 tsp chili powder
- 1 tsp cumin
- 1/2 tsp oregano
- Salt and pepper to taste
- Chopped cilantro for garnish (optional)

Instructions:

1. In a large skillet over medium•high heat, cook the ground beef until browned and crumbled, 5•7 minutes. Drain any excess fat.

2. Add the quinoa and beef broth to the skillet. Bring to a boil, then reduce heat to low, cover and simmer for 15•20 minutes, until quinoa is cooked through.

3. Stir in the diced tomatoes, bell pepper, onion, garlic, chili powder, cumin and oregano. Season with salt and pepper to taste.

4. Cook for an additional 5 minutes, until vegetables are tender.

5. Serve the beef and quinoa mixture in bowls, garnished with chopped cilantro if desired.

This makes a hearty, protein•packed meal that's easy to prepare. The quinoa adds fiber and nutrients, while the beef provides satisfying protein. Feel free to customize the vegetables to your liking.

Congratulations on completing the *"Weight Loss Muscle Gain Cookbook: Macro Friendly Grab & Burn Fat, Build Muscles, Low, Medium, High Carb Days."* By exploring the recipes and meal plans within these pages, you have taken a significant step toward achieving your fitness and nutritional goals. This journey is more than just about losing weight or gaining muscle—it's about adopting a sustainable, balanced approach to eating that enhances your overall well-being.

Reflecting on Your Journey

As you reflect on the delicious meals and new habits you've developed, remember that the principles of macro-friendly eating and carb cycling are tools you can carry forward. These concepts empower you to tailor your diet to your unique needs, supporting your body through various phases of activity and rest. By understanding and implementing these strategies, you've equipped yourself with the knowledge to maintain and even surpass your health goals.

Sustaining Your Success

Consistency is key to long-term success. Continue to experiment with the recipes, adjust your meal plans according to your progress, and embrace the flexibility that comes with a macro-friendly approach. Remember that it's normal to have fluctuations and that each meal is an opportunity to nourish your body and mind.

Expanding Your Horizons

Don't hesitate to expand your culinary repertoire beyond the recipes provided here. Use the principles learned in this cookbook to create your own dishes that fit your macro needs and taste preferences. Share your journey with others, inspire them with your progress, and perhaps even collaborate on new recipes and meal plans.

A Lifelong Commitment

Health and fitness are lifelong commitments. The knowledge and skills you've gained from this cookbook are the foundation upon which you can build a lifetime of healthy eating and active living. Stay curious, stay motivated, and most importantly, stay kind to yourself. Progress is not always linear, and every step forward, no matter how small, is a victory.

Here's to your health, your strength, and your continued success. Enjoy the journey and savor every moment of it!